SPORTS AND ATHLETICS PREPARATION, PERFORMANCE,
AND PSYCHOLOGY

PERSPECTIVES ON ANABOLIC ANDROGENIC STEROIDS (AAS) AND DOPING IN SPORT AND HEALTH

SPORTS AND ATHLETICS PREPARATION, PERFORMANCE, AND PSYCHOLOGY

SUBSTANCE ABUSE ASSESSMENT, INTERVENTIONS AND TREATMENT

SPORTS AND ATHLETICS PREPARATION, PERFORMANCE, AND PSYCHOLOGY

PERSPECTIVES ON ANABOLIC ANDROGENIC STEROIDS (AAS) AND DOPING IN SPORT AND HEALTH

FERGAL GRACE

AND

JULIEN S. BAKER

EDITORS

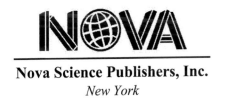

Nova Science Publishers, Inc.

New York

LIBRARY OF CONGRESS CATALOGING-IN-PUBLICATION DATA

Perspectives on anabolic androgenic steroids (AAS) and doping in sport and health / [edited by] Fergal Grace and Julien S. Baker.
  p. cm.
Includes index.
ISBN 978-1-62081-243-3 (hardcover)
1. Anabolic steroids--Health aspects. 2. Doping in sports. I. Grace, Fergal. II. Baker, Julien.
RC1230.P4785 2011
362.29--dc23
                    2012006536

Published by Nova Science Publishers, Inc. † *New York*

CONTENTS

PREFACE

Anabolic androgenic steroids (AAS) remain the most used/abused drugs in the athlete and recreational gym user. However, there are some new drugs such as human growth hormone and insulin that are being used by athletes in order to gain a competitive advantage. This book presents separate and multi-disciplinary perspectives of anabolic androgenic steroids and other current drugs of use in sport. The perspectives discussed in this book range from those of sports medicine research scientists, a medical practitioner and sports physician, behavioral scientists and molecular physiologists. There are further contributions from experts in the sociology and ethics of sports doping.

Chapter 1 - The use of doping agents by individuals involved in sports is not decreasing. Anabolic-androgenic steroids (AAS) or 'anabolic steroids' remain the most widely abused drugs. Such drugs can have serious physiological and psychological effects, which should preclude their abuse. The escalation of drug taking in this market has also predisposed opportunities for counterfeiting, with the consequences of adverse effects from non-sterile contamination causing a variety of communicable diseases and other health problems throughout the world of sport. The law is currently vascillatory. In the USA, possession is a federal offence, but it is not in the UK or Europe. However, it is illegal to take drugs in all professional sports with the exception of bodybuilding, where no testing is currently conducted.

The majority of dope testing that is conducted is in the field of athletics, in individual sporting events. Team sports have enjoyed a sustained degree of immunity. The consensus of opinion is that the team player would be less likely to wish to bring disrepute on their compatriots, but it is often suggested that team sports (such as football) are more powerful as an industry, than the authorities that test them. Counterfeiting markets have dominated the field of drug use to such an extent that immense temptation pervades for succumbing to the lures of fame and fortune that derive from sporting success. The policy of 'zero tolerance' has failed. Management of this dilemma needs to achieved through education.

Chapter 2 - Androgen endocrine physiology is responsible for many processes in the body, from bone metabolism to skeletal muscle maintenance. Testosterone (T) is one of the most potent androgens produced, with decades of research highlighting its androgenic-anabolic effect on skeletal muscle growth. The research has been further driven through the emergence of pharmaceutical derivates (steroids) of T and their use in interventions for muscle wasting associated with disease and advancing age (sarcopenia). However, the molecular regulation of T and the influence it has on cellular processes in promoting muscle development, hypertrophy and satellite cell activation (proliferation, differentiation) remain poorly understood. The utilisation of human, animal models and cell culture have begun to suggest the molecular mechanisms by which T acts on skeletal muscle, yet often the results remain inconclusive. This review therefore highlights the most current research into the molecular mechanisms of T with suggested future direction. An emergent feature is the possible lack of biomimicity between monolayer cell culture models and the *in-vivo* environment. Bio-engineered skeletal muscle thus represents a physiological tool to bridge the gap by incorporating a native cell niche and extracellular environment that skeletal muscle has *in-vivo*. With future experimentation and by unravelling key cellular and molecular mechanisms of testosterone regulation there is the potential to harness the un-refutable power of this hormone in order to implement interventions for sarcopenia and muscle wasting diseases.

Chapter 3 - This chapter reflects the thought and concerns of a general practitioner and sports physician in relation to the use of anabolic androgenic steroids (AAS). Colleagues in general practice associate their use with the sport of weightlifting, wrestling and bodybuilding in the main. This chapter will summarise the currently available information on AAS use by the sports person and centres on who is using them, reasons for use, supplementation regimens and associated side effects which commonly present at sports clinic and general practice.

Chapter 4 - Studies investigating the effects of Anabolic Androgenic Steroids (AAS) on the cardiovascular system have been present in the medical literature over the past forty years. The present chapter reviews the available literature on the impact that AAS use has on cardiovascular structure and function from the more popular studies in the 1980s, investigating the effects of AAS on cholesterol levels to the more currently popular studies that aim to identify the underlying mechanisms behind remodeling of cardiac muscle. There is currently good progress being made in understanding the physiological mechanisms behind AAS induced cardio-toxicity from both the in vitro and animal model. If current rates of progress are continued and the medical research community continues to publish both controlled and case studies then a clearer understanding of the mechanisms behind cardiovascular problems resulting from AAS use are expected in the near future.

Chapter 5 - Anabolic-androgenic steroids (AAS) is the broad term used to describe the male sex hormone testosterone and other endogenous androgenic hormones. It is also an expression used for synthesised products of these hormones. The male sex hormone testosterone is primarily responsible for anabolic and androgenic effects highlighted in male childhood and adolescence. AAS can be used legally, for example, prescribed as a treatment for delayed puberty and for conditions that may result in muscle wasting. There is however, significant concern at the non-prescribed use of these products and the use of these hormones in this context will be the primary focus of this chapter.

Synthetic products of testosterone occurred shortly after it was initially isolated in the 1930s. Anabolic means simply to encourage tissue growth by increasing the metabolic process. Androgen is described as a group of steroid hormones that includes testosterone and dihydrotestosterone. The most abundant androgen is testosterone with 95% being secreted by the testicular Leydig cells. In addition to testosterone, the testes also secrete small amounts of the weak androgens droepiandrosterone and androstenedione.

The main source of these hormones is the testes. The hormones are responsible for male sexual features such as beard growth, deep voice and muscle development. Anabolic steroids are synthetic forms of male hormones which include the drug nandrolone. Supraphysiologic doses of AAS combined with arduous exercise and good nutrition can cause users to unnaturally gain body muscle. Nevertheless, the precise biological mechanisms responsible for these transformations remain unclear.

Chapter 6 - This chapter presents a sociological investigation into the perceptions of, and opinions about those involved in elite level sports concerning the use performance enhancing drugs. An interpretivist approach was adopted that sought to highlight the real life experiences of key stake-holders from the elite level of one particular high-profile, multi-event sport. The 'sociological voices' were crafted into non-fictional narratives and include contributions from an international competitor inexperienced at senior level, three Olympians, a Paralympian, an elite level specialist coach, and a senior administrator – of these, two were female. The data are presented in this way to synthesise the findings into an accessible form, and protect the anonymity of those involved. The main themes to emerge from the interviews and presented in the narratives include: the pressures and responsibilities of being an elite performer, the relation of performance to financial security, the fairness and integrity of sports, the perception of variable robustness of testing amongst different countries, differences between junior level and senior competition and between men and women.

Chapter 7 - The aim of this chapter is to offer a consideration of philosophical and ethical arguments that are grounded in the contexts of anabolic androgenic steroid (AAS) use and doping in sports participation. Sports may be seen as an unusual family of social practices that, while aiming at excellence, delimits the legitimate ways in which participants may prepare for, and perform in, those social practices. The present chapter sketches the terrain within the academic bioethics literature concerning the use of AAS for therapy and enhancement. There is examination as to the extent of the prevalence of AAS use within the sporting environment including the standard arguments that are raised within the philosophy of sports ethics giving consideration to the specific policy position of the World Anti Doping Agency (WADA).

Chapter 8 - Athletes are taking growth hormone and insulin, separately or in combination with the intention of increasing skeletal muscle mass hoping to improve performance and there is powerful scientific evidence to suggest this is possible. Adding some insulin-like growth factor, for example, Epo and myostatin inhibitor to the mixture and an almost undetectable cocktail is created that can promote significant muscle growth. Each of these drugs is on the World Anti-Doping Agency's (WADA's) banned list. However, if they are cycled correctly and unless an athlete is caught in possession of the drugs or tested within 24 hours of administration, the opportunity of proving a case of doping diminishes exponentially. There appears to be little problem obtaining such agents. These elixirs are not for sale from local superstores, but from unlicensed laboratories, to which the Internet has given *bona fide* credibility and a medium for conveyance.

In: Perspectives on Anabolic Androgenic ....   ISBN: 978-1-62081-243-3
Editors: F. Grace and J. S. Baker   © 2012 Nova Science Publishers, Inc.

Chapter 1

ANABOLIC STEROIDS USED AS DOPING AGENTS IN SPORTS

Michael Graham[1,], Peter Evans[2] and Bruce Davies[3]*

[1]Sport and Exercise Science, Institute of Health, Medical Science and
Society Science, Glyndwr University, Wrexham, Wales, UK
[2]Dept Diabetes and Endocrinology, Royal Gwent Hospital, Newport,
Gwent, Wales, UK
[3]Dept of Health and Exercise Science, University of Glamorgan,
Mid Glamorgan. Wales, UK

ABSTRACT

The use of doping agents by individuals involved in sports is not
decreasing. Anabolic-androgenic steroids (AAS) or 'anabolic steroids'
remain the most widely abused drugs. Such drugs can have serious
physiological and psychological effects, which should preclude their
abuse. The escalation of drug taking in this market has also predisposed
opportunities for counterfeiting, with the consequences of adverse effects
from non-sterile contamination causing a variety of communicable
diseases and other health problems throughout the world of sport. The
law is currently vascillatory. In the USA, possession is a federal offence,
but it is not in the UK or Europe. However, it is illegal to take drugs in all
professional sports with the exception of bodybuilding, where no testing
is currently conducted.

---

* Email: m.graham@glyndwr.ac.uk.

The majority of dope testing that is conducted is in the field of athletics, in individual sporting events. Team sports have enjoyed a sustained degree of immunity. The consensus of opinion is that the team player would be less likely to wish to bring disrepute on their compatriots, but it is often suggested that team sports (such as football) are more powerful as an industry, than the authorities that test them. Counterfeiting markets have dominated the field of drug use to such an extent that immense temptation pervades for succumbing to the lures of fame and fortune that derive from sporting success. The policy of 'zero tolerance' has failed. Management of this dilemma needs to achieved through education.

BIOCHEMISTRY AND PHYSIOLOGY

The hormone, *Testosterone* was first isolated from testicles in May 1935 by David and colleagues [1] working for the pharmaceutical company Organon, in Holland. Its structure was determined by Butenandt working for the pharmaceutical company Schering in Germany [2] and first synthesized from cholesterol in August, 1935 [3]. One week later, when working for the pharmaceutical company Ciba in Zurich, Switzerland, Ruzicka also published the synthesis of testosterone [4] These independent syntheses of testosterone, to replace deficiency, earned both Butenandt and Ruzicka the joint Nobel Prize in Chemistry, in 1939.

Testosterone was identified as 17β-hydroxyandrost-4-en-3-one ($C_{19}H_{28}O_2$), a solid polycyclic alcohol with a hydroxyl group at the 17th carbon atom (Figure 1). This made it obvious that additional modifications on the synthesized testosterone could be made, i.e., esterification and alkylation (Figure 2). In the mid 1930s the synthesis of potent testosterone esters identified the characterisation of the hormones effects, that testosterone raised nitrogen retention (a mechanism central to anabolism) after which both anabolic and androgenic effects of testosterone propionate in boys, eunuchs and women could be demonstrated [5].

Today the terms androgenic-anabolic steroid (AAS) or anabolic steroids refer to a group of synthetic compounds similar in chemical structure to the natural male steroid hormone testosterone and dihydrotestosterone (DHT) [6]. Male steroid hormones, primarily testosterone, are partially responsible for the developmental changes that occur during adolescence. Testosterone concentrations in the blood are controlled by a negative feedback system from the hypothalamic-pituitary-gonadal axis.

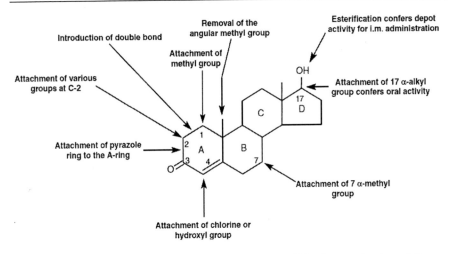

Figure 1. The structure of testosterone and structural modifications to the A- and B-rings of this steroid molecule that increase anabolic activity. Substitution at C-17 confers oral or depot activity, IM = intramuscular (Reproduced with permission from kicman and Gower, 2003 [70].

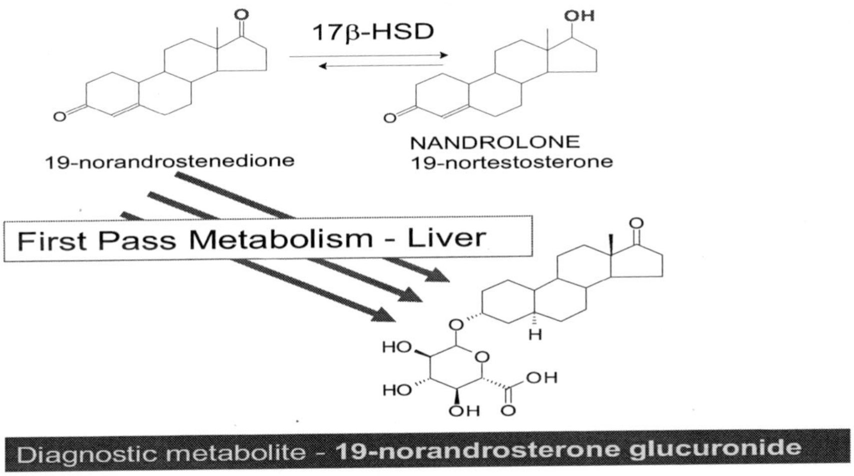

17β-HSD

19-norandrostenedione

NANDROLONE
19-nortestosterone

First Pass Metabolism - Liver

Diagnostic metabolite - **19-norandrosterone glucuronide**

Figure 2. Nandrolone and its diagnostic metabolites. In androgenic tissues 19-nortestosterone is converted by the enzyme 5α-reductase into the metabolite "5α-dihydro-19-nortestosterone". This binds with a weaker affinity to the androgen receptor (AR) compared with the parent steroid so further metabolism can occur. In anabolic tissue (skeletal muscle) 5α-reductase activity is negligible, so the parent steroid binds with high affinity to the AR. Therefore there is increased anabolic (myotrophic)-to-androgenic activity compared to the natural testosterone molecule.

In normal males there are some individual differences in the daily quantity of testosterone produced (usually 6-10 mg.day^{-1}). It is synthesised by the interstitial Leydig cells of the testes, primarily under control of the gonadotrophins secreted by the pituitary gland.

Approximately 95% of circulating testosterone originates directly from testicular secretion [4]. Following secretion, testosterone is then transported via the blood to target organs and specific receptor sites. Several bodily functions are under direct or indirect control of testosterone.

Testosterone, the predominant circulating testicular androgen, is both an active hormone and a prohormone for the formation of a more active androgen, the 5 α-reduced steroid, DHT. Physiological studies of steroid hormone metabolism in the postnatal state demonstrate that DHT is formed in target tissues from circulating testosterone and is a more potent androgen than testosterone in several bioassay systems [7].

Genetic evidence indicates that these two androgens work via a common intracellular receptor. The androgen receptor (AR) is an intracellular ligand-dependent protein which modulates the expression of genes and mediates biological actions of physiological androgens (testosterone and 5 α- DHT) in a cell-specific manner [8].

During embryonic life, androgens cause the formation of the male urogenital tract and hence are responsible for development of the tissues that serve as the major sites of androgen action in postnatal life. It has been generally assumed that androgens virilise the male foetus by the same mechanisms as in the adult, namely by the conversion of circulating testosterone to DHT in target tissues.

DHT binds to the AR more tightly than testosterone, primarily as a result of stabilisation of the AR complex and at low concentrations, is as effective as testosterone at high concentrations in enhancing the transcription of one response element [9].

This finding clearly indicates that some effects of DHT are the result of amplification of the testosterone signal. DHT formation acts both as a general amplifier of androgen action and conveys specific function to the androgen-AR complex.

The enzyme aromatase controls the androgen/oestrogen ratio by catalysing the conversion of testosterone into oestradiol (E2). Therefore, the regulation of E2 synthesis by aromatase is thought to be critical in sexual development and differentiation [10].

AAS AND SPORT

Sports men and women use AAS to improve muscle mass and strength [11] with the intention of enhancing performance, but they also take them for cosmetic reasons to improve image [12] Their use can cause physiological and psychological dependence [13] and adverse cardiovascular effects [14] The bodily functions which are under direct control of testosterone that have relevance to the athlete can be divided into two broad classifications: male hormonal effects (androgenic functions) and constructive or muscle building effects (anabolic functions). The balance between androgenic and anabolic functions differ in each steroid hormone, but there is no AAS that has an anabolic effect in an athlete without an androgenic effect [15].

AAS have had therapeutic uses in the past. Testosterone tends to be more androgenic than anabolic, therefore chemical modification of the basic testosterone molecule has formed the basis for the clinical application of synthetic AAS. Pharmaceutical companies initially developed these synthetic analogues of testosterone in order to treat catabolic medical conditions, such as androgen deficiency, osteoporosis, chronic obstructive pulmonary disease, burns and human immunodeficiency [16]. Nandrolone one of the most anabolic derivatives of testosterone, was initially used in disseminated metastatic carcinoma of the breast (Figure 2). AAS are still currently the most commonly used group of drugs used in competitive sport, despite advances in detection techniques and severe reprisals for testing positive.

LEGAL ASPECTS SURROUNDING AAS USE

AAS are controlled substances in several countries, including Australia, Argentina, Brazil, Canada, the UK and the USA. Despite this, there is a readily available worldwide supply of AAS, for non-medicinal purposes. In many countries, AAS can be sold legally without a prescription [17;18] Consequently, many foreign distributors do not violate the laws of their own country when they sell these substances to customers overseas, whether directly via the Internet or e-mail orders. Similarly recipients of such substances in the UK do not contravene national laws if they are for personal use. The majority of the hormonal products in the European market come from countries within the European Union, but also from Thailand, Turkey, Egypt, India and Pakistan [18].

Table 1. Intramuscular (IM) AAS analysed by GC-MS. Products were provided by bodybuilders. Transdermal AAS Patches analysed by GC-MS. Products were obtained from popular bodybuilding website. Products either did not contain what was stated on the label, or contained no active ingredient

	Product label	Ingredients claimed	Active ingredients found
1	BOLDENONA 50	BOLDENONE UNDECYLENATE	TESTOSTERONE PROPIONATE
2	NANDROLONE DECANOATE	NANDROLONE DECANOATE	TESTOSTERONE ENANTHATE
3	PRIMOBOLAN DEPOT	METHENOLONE ENANTHATE	NANDROLONE PHENYLPROPIONATE
4	SUSTANON	TESTOSTERONE PROPIONATE, TESTOSTERONE PHENYLPROPIONATE, TESTOSTERONE ISOCAPROATE, TESTOSTERONE DECANOATE	TESTOSTERONE PROPIONATE, TESTOSTERONE PHENYLPROPIONATE TESTOSTERONE DECANOATE, TESTOSTERONE ENANTHATE
5	TRENBOLONE 80	TRENBOLONE ENANTHATE	TRENBOLONE ACETATE
6	SACHET 1	WWW.821.IN "TEP, 3 ML"	TESTOSTERONE PROPIONATE
7	SACHET 2	WWW.821.IN "INDIAN AROMATHERAPY OILS, TE3, 3 ML"	TESTOSTERONE PROPIONATE, TESTOSTERONE CYPIONATE, TESTOSTERONE DECANOATE
8	BOLDABOL	BOLDENONE UNDECYLENATE	NOTHING
9	BOLDEBAL-H	BOLDENONE UNDECYLENATE	NOTHING
10	MASTABOL	DROMASTANOLONE DIPROPIONATE	NOTHING
11	PRIMOBOLAN DEPOT	METHENOLONE ENANTHATE	NOTHING
12	SPECTRIOL	TESTOSTERONE ESTERS	NOTHING
13	TESTABOL DEPOT	TESTOSTERONE CYPIONATE	NOTHING
14	TESTEX ELMU PROLANGATUM 250	TESTOSTERONE CYPIONATE	NOTHING
15	TESOSTERONE CYPIONATE INJECTION (CYPIONAX)	TESTOSTERONE CYPIONATE	NOTHING
16	TRENBOL 75-R	TRENBOLONE ACETATE	NOTHING

In the USA, significant quantities of anabolic steroids come from Mexico, as well as other countries such as Russia, Romania, and Greece [17]. With the development of capital expansion in less developed countries and their use of economical manual labour and the Internet revolution the availability of these drugs has become available at the touch of a computer button and the use of a credit card.

Since 1996 in the UK, AAS are controlled under Schedule IV (Part II) of the Misuse of Drugs Act. There is no restriction on the possession of these substances when they are part of a medicinal product and are for self-administration. However, as a consequence of their controlled legal status in the UK, AAS are frequently obtained from sources of unknown provenance, such as the black market or by using the Internet. Such products are not subjected to the level of scrutiny of standardised quality assurance for prescription medicines that are obtained through legitimate sources.

AAS AND TRANSMISSION OF INFECTION

The increase in 'performance and image enhancing drugs' (PIEDs) has led to several assessments and analyses of the type of drugs being used. *Table 1* identifies one cache of anabolic steroids, which were shown to be counterfeit.

Outbreaks of intramuscular (IM) abscesses in bodybuilders, thought to be as a result of the use of non-sterilised or contaminated counterfeit products has recently demonstrated this level of counterfeit products available from the black market [19] Forty three percent of all samples were shown to be counterfeit and microbiological culture of drug samples revealed the presence of skin commensals which in an inappropriate environment can function as pathological contaminants. Populations of microbes (such as bacteria and yeasts) inhabit the skin and mucosa. Their role forms part of normal, healthy human physiology, however if microbe numbers grow beyond their typical ranges (often due to a compromised immune system) or if microbes populate atypical areas of the body (such as through poor hygiene, injury or needle transmission), acute and chronic infections can result.

Prevalence of use continues despite increased educational programmes. In 2001, 69% of respondents of hardcore gym weight-lifters, were identified as abusing AAS [20] A survey conducted by Parkinson and Evans in 2006 [21] estimated that steroids are being abused by more than 3 million Americans. A survey undertaken in the South Wales area found that 70% of respondents were regular AAS users and 7% were females and estimated that they are being abused by more than 1 million UK citizens, with unsafe injection practices, such as reusing and sharing needles and multidose vials [22; 23].

The abuse of AAS by females corresponds with the same rationale of abuse of AAS by males. They are taken for cosmetic purposes, to increase muscle mass and to minimise fat mass. The administration of AAS in males is often driven by illogical and unscientific peer-pressure. Multiple doses of the same drug, which have different labels, but are different brand names of the same product, are often taken under the assumption that they will have a greater effect on muscular development. Such myths contradict current scientific research, which has shown that there is only one testosterone receptor [24]. Polypharmacy is another problem that is encountered, different drugs being taken to counteract the occurrence of adverse side effects. Males use tamoxifen to counteract the aromatisation of excess testosterone, which can lead to gynaecomastia [25]. Female bodybuilders also self-prescribe tamoxifen, despite it being an oestrogen receptor antagonist. There would appear to be no logical explanation for a female taking tamoxifen, an aromatase inhibitor, used medically as a treatment for carcinoma of the breast, however, female bodybuilders have claimed tamoxifen prevents breast discomfort. Administration of large volumes of testosterone esters in one injection (up to 5 mls) is not uncommon.

Injection practices can place an individual at risk of a sterile abscess, where a pathogenic organism is not found, following surgical evacuation [26] [27] identified that 50% of bodybuilders were administering their drugs IM and that non-sterile technique, reported sharing of AAS multidosage vials was placing them at risk of IM abscesses. Reported infections associated with AAS injection include abscesses attributable to Mycobacterium Smegmatis, Staphylococcus, Streptococcus, Pseudomonas, Hepatitis B, Hepatitis C and human immunodeficiency virus [28]. Thigh abscesses, gluteal, pectoral and deltoid abscess have been reported in bodybuilders using 'site locations', which are local injections into a specific muscle, believed to increase isolated muscle growth [29].

PUBLIC HEALTH ISSUE

In America in the 1980s, government policies were developed to curtail AAS use. These policies decreased the production of AAS by domestic pharmaceutical companies and lowered their availability to recreational users. The resulting demand was filled by a counterfeit market. These counterfeiters could not be scrutinised by the Food and Drug Administration (FDA) which often produce their drugs in non-sterile conditions. This unregulated manufacture has produced steroid preparations that have been contaminated with infectious agents and are of poor quality [30].

In the UK, the counterfeiting market has led to the sale and distribution of large quantities of multidosage vials. Their use is indirectly encouraged by the expense of AAS preparations and is a common practice among bodybuilders. Many users purchase a vial together and share its contents. Contamination of vials with used needles is an effective vehicle to transmit blood-borne pathogens [31] This is comparable to the sharing of spoons among intravenous drug users, who inject recreational street drugs [32]. Education and the unquestioned provision of "once-only use" of sterile needles remains a practical way to prevent abscesses and blood borne infections for such individuals. Needle exchange programs currently provide AAS users with clean, sterile needles and may be a unique opportunity for intervention and education to this population [33].

Despite the provision of sterile needles and syringes to user groups, there has been a pandemic increase in Hepatitis C virus (HCV), in recreational drug abuse. It has a global prevalence of 3%, causing chronic infection in 75% of cases, and is currently the main cause of liver transplant in the United Kingdom [34] Globally, 50% of the population of recreational drug users are suffering with HCV [35] and in the USA a conservative estimate is that 5.2 million individuals are also infected [36]. The strongest factor independently associated with HCV infection is illegal drug use. AAS which are being taken as PIEDs are increasing within the health and fitness industry, especially in females [23] with a corresponding increase in communicable diseases in this population also. Legislature does not appear to have curtailed the growth of this industry, but hopefully prevention by education and the unlimited provision of sterile equipment with the assurance of anonymity, appears to be the way to combat escalation [37].

ASSOCIATION BETWEEN DOPING, SCIENCE AND SPORT

The involvement of sports medicine practitioners in elite sport has concerned them in the quest for championship-winning and record-breaking performances. This has led them not only to develop improved nutrition, or mechanical and psychological techniques (ergogenic aids) but, to a significant extent, to be implicated in the development and use of performance enhancing drugs. Sport's physicians were involved in the state-sponsored systematic doping of athletes in the former East Germany [38; 39] American Sports Scientists have also been implicated in the dissemination of performance and image enhancing drugs used in international sport. Ziegler, an American physician, originally developed the anabolic steroid Methandrostenolone (Dianabol) which was released in the USA in 1958 by Ciba. He pioneered its athletic use as an aid to muscle growth by bodybuilders, administering it to USA weightlifting champion Bill March of the York Barbell club in 1959 when he was the physician to the USA Weightlifting team. This was thought to be the first use of AAS in sport [40]. The network of relationships between those involved in purchasing, and supplying drugs in sport has been extensive. The emphasis and rewards placed on winning and breaking world records has made this liaison between sporting performance and sports science almost inextricable.

PUBLIC ENQUIRIES INTO AAS ABUSE

Prior to the 'Dubin Inquiry' in 1990, the attention in doping cases was upon an athlete who tested positive [41] No effort was made to ascertain if the doctors, coaches, or trainers were involved in such collusion [38]. Past confessions from sprint athletes, such as; Ben Johnson, Kelly White, Tim Montgomery, Marion Jones and the UK athlete Dwain Chambers have demonstrated that they were prepared to tread the fine lines that separated success from failure.

Rewards are so vast, that anonymous surveys have identified that elite athletes will risk ill health, and even premature death, if they believe they can cheat, win and not get caught [42]. The USA Federal investigation into the the Bay Area Laboratory Co-operative (BALCO) in the provision of 'designer steroids' such as Tetrahydrogestrinone (THG) coded as 'The Clear', which can be ingested sublingually and was supplied to high profile athletes, such as Dwain Chambers [43]. The BALCO affair, attracted media attention not least because of the supply of THG but also the supply of a transdermal preparation, 'The Cream', that contained testosterone (T) and epitestosterone (E), produced specifically to evade a doping T/E ratio urinalysis. The "Mitchell Report" has provided us with some of the clues that have lead to this unholy alliance [44]. It covers the history of the use of illegal performance-enhancing substances by players in the Major League Baseball.

Table 2. Adverse side effects of AAS administration in order of severity.
The adverse side effects and potential dangers of AAS abuse are well
documented [45]

Organ	Side Effect	Result
Cardiovascular System	Dyslipidaemia; distortion of clotting factors; cardiac ventricular hypertrophy	Cerebrovascular accident (stroke) or myocardial infarction (heart attack) leading to sudden death
Central Nervous System	Psychological and Psychiatric effects	Euphoria Depression Increased aggression Increased or Decreased Libido Psychosis
Hepato-Portal System (Liver-Gall Bladder-Spleen)	Peliosis hepatis (Liver cysts); cholestatic (obstructive) jaundice; Liver tumours (cancer); distorted Liver enzymes	Ruptured Liver cysts leading to peritonitis. Cholecystitis leading to peritonitis. Malignant Liver tumours can metastasise (spread to other organs).
Reproductive System	Distortion of gonadal steroidogenesis; Males - testicular atrophy; prostatic hypertrophy; breast pain; gynaecomastia. Females – clitoral hypertrophy, breast pain; breast atrophy	Infertility. Some AAS are aromatised more than others, requiring the use of oestrogen receptor antagonists (tamoxifen/anastrozole) or corrective surgery. Virilisation of the female foetus (shemale).
Skeletal System	Premature closure of epiphyses in children	Restriction of linear growth (ultimate height).
Skin	Acne Vulgaris Acne Rosacea Cystic Acne Abscesses	Can be initiated or exacerbated, causing extensive scarring and requiring medical and surgical intervention and leading to psychological and psychiatric sequelae.
Hair	Males and females– Initiation or exacerbation of baldness. Females - Hirsutism	Can be irreversible
Larynx	Hypertrophy	Can be irreversible
Intramuscular Injection sites (Skin and muscle)	Abscesses; Bacteria Viruses	Abscesses requiring medical and surgical intervention. Viruses - Hepatitis B, C, Human Immunodeficiency Virus (HIV)

AAS and the Olympics: AAS were the first identified doping agents to be banned in sport, by the International Olympic Committee (IOC) Medical Commission, in Athens in 1961. At this time the political medical opinion of the day disputed that AAS had any effect on muscle development in adult males. It was accepted that they had effect in adult males with hypothalamic-hypogonadism, children and females but it wasn't until 1996 when computerised scanning proved indisputably that they increase muscle mass and strength and could enhance physical performance and improve appearance [11].

There are four types of AAS used by athletes, based on the route of administration by the athlete or the carrier solvent: 1. Oral AAS preparations; 2. Injectable AAS preparations; 3. Transdermal AAS preparations; 4. Sublingual AAS preparations.

Oral AAS are synthesised in order to offer protection to the molecule when it becomes exposed to the strong acid solutions found in the stomach, and when it contacts the liver's enzymic mechanisms. Oral activity is conferred by the substitution of a methyl (CH_3) or ethyl (C_2H_5) group for H on the carbon atom (C) on the cyclopentane ring structure, in position 17 (C-17). The 17α-alkylated steroids prevent deactivation by the first-pass metabolism by sterically hindering oxidation of the 17 β-hydroxyl group. Liver dysfunction has been recorded as a consequence of chronic abuse, longer than 6 months, but probably in excessive dosages [46]. The treatment of hereditary angioedema patients with therapeutic oral stanozolol or danazol did not cause adverse hepatic changes [47]. Oral activity can also be conferred by attachment of a methyl group at C-1 as in methenolone or mesterolone, but the potency of the steroid is far weaker.

There are weaker formulations of anabolic agents which have the classification of "nutritional" or "dietary" supplements and are marketed as "pro-hormones": dehydroepiandrosterone (DHEA), androstenedione, 19-norandrostenedione, androstenediol and 19-norandrostenediol. These "steroids", or "sterols" of plant extract, lack the 17α-alkyl moiety and are extensively metabolised by the liver on the first pass metabolism. DHEA and androstenedione do not bind to the AR, but they are substrates, used by the adrenal glands and converted to testosterone and thus may have a weak androgenic effect. Androstenediol has been shown to activate AR target genes in the presence of AR [48].

Little research has been done on 19-norandrostenedione and 19-norandrostenediol, but as a consequence of high profile drug doping offences, in athletes, 19-norandrostenedione was made a controlled drug, in the UK.

Characteristics of oral preparations:

1. They have a structure that acidic gastric secretions of the stomach will not render ineffective by degradation.

2. They have the capability to be absorbed into the gastrointestinal tract, usually the stomach or the proximal small bowel.
3. They are able to withstand total degradation by the liver enzymes.
4. They have a short half live. In order to maintain the appropriate blood concentration the drug must be taken several times a day.
5. Following the initial pass through the liver the drug must still retain the capacity to bind with the AR sites present in skeletal muscle.

Injectable preparations do not require a 17 α-alkyl group but the 17 β-hydroxyl group is esterified with an acid moiety to prevent rapid absorption from the oily vehicle which is usually arachis oil and benzyl alcohol [49].
Characteristics of injectable oil based preparations are:

1. They have a much longer half-life than oral or water based injectable steroids, usually in the order of 1-4 weeks.
2. They are normally comprised of a mixture of arachis/sesame seed oil and alcohol which forms the basis of the oil based carrier.
3. The concentration of AAS esters range from 25 to 250 mg.ml-1, per dosage.
4. They have a degree of pain at the injection site.
5. They have a slow absorption rate into the blood stream, so that the liver experiences a low concentration of the drug compared to substances taken orally. This may be associated with less incidence of liver disorder than that associated with oral preparations [50].
6. Basic alteration of the steroid ring at the 17-β, will prolong the effect of the drug.

Characteristics of injectable water based steroids are:

1. They have a half life of 1-2 weeks, therefore they require more frequent injections.
2. They have less discomfort at the injection site because of a lower viscosity compared to the same oil-based anabolic agent.
3. They have a molecular structure that is in most cases identical to oil based preparations.
4. They have the ability to mix with other water based anabolic steroids or water based vitamins e.g. B12 [51].

METHODS OF AAS ADMINISTRATION IN SPORT

Personal communications with AAS users has highlighted the following non-scientific methods of use:

1. *Stacking/Blending/Shot-gunning*: Using more than one drug at the same time. Individuals frequently use several anabolic steroids simultaneously, mixing oral and/or injectable types, sometimes using drugs such as stimulants or painkillers.
   The rationale for stacking is a belief-which has not been tested scientifically, that different drugs have a synergistic effect on muscle size.
2. *Tapering*: Gradually decreasing intake.
   Plateauing: When a drug becomes ineffective at a particular level another drug is taken.
3. *Cycling*: Using different drugs for a fixed period usually 6-12 weeks, cessation of administration for the same period of time, and then repeating the cycle.
4. *Pyramiding*: Maximising dosage within a fixed space of time and then minimising the drug in the same time frame.

Table 3. Typical AAS Regime of a first time user. (Personal communications with a current UK champion)

Week	1	2	3	4	5	6	7	8	9	10	11	12
Drug	Dose											
Sustanon (IM) (250 mg.ml^{-1}.week^{-1})	1	1	1	1								
methandienone (5 mg.tablet^{-1}.d^{-1}) (oral)	6	6	6	6	6	6	6	6	6	6	6	6
nandrolone decanoate (IM) (100 mg.ml^{-1}.week^{-1})				2	2	2	2	2				
stanozolol suspension (IM) (50 mg.ml^{-1}.week^{-1})									3	3	3	3

IM = Intramuscular (parenteral) administration;
d^{-1} = daily dose; week^{-1}= weekly dose.

Table 4. AAS Regime of a UK champion (Personal communications)

Week	16	15	14	13	12	11	10	9	8	7	6	5	4	3	2	1
Drug	Dose															
Omnadren (IM) (250 mg.ml^{-1}.week^{-1})	2	2	1	1	1	2										
testosterone enanthate (250 mg.ml^{-1}.week^{-1}) (IM)			1	1	1	1										
nandrolone decanoate (100 mg.ml^{-1}.week^{-1}) (IM)	2	2	2	2	2	2										
methandienone (5 mg.tablet^{-1}.d^{-1}) (oral)	10	10	10	10	10	8	6	4								
Sustanon (IM) (250 mg.ml^{-1}.week^{-1})				1												
testosterone propionate (IM) (100 mg.ml^{-1}.week^{-1})													4	4	4	4
(testosterone cypionate) (IM) (250 mg.ml^{-1}.week^{-1})								2	2	2	2	6	6	6	6	4
mesterelone (oral) (25 mg.tablet^{-1}.d^{-1})											1	1	1	2	2	2
growth hormone (Somatropin) (SC) (IU.d^{-1})								2.5	2.5	2.5	5	5	10	10	10	
clomiphene citrate (50 mg.tablet^{-1}.d^{-1}) (oral)								0.5	0.5	0.5	0.5	0.5				
tamoxifen (oral) (20 mg.tablet^{-1}.d^{-1})	1	1	1	1	1	1	1	1	1	1	1	1	2	3		
clenbuterol (20 µg.tablet^{-1}.d^{-1}) (oral)								5	5	5	5	5	5	5	5	5
stanozolol suspension (50 mg.ml^{-1}.week^{-1}) (IM)											3	4	5	4	4	3
anastrazole (1 mg.tablet^{-1}.d^{-1}) (oral)													1	1	1	1
methenolone enanthate (100 mg.ml^{-1}.week^{-1}) (IM)											3	3	3	3	3	3
aminoglutethimide (250 mg.tablet^{-1}.d^{-1})(oral)														1	1	1

Table 4. (Continued)

Week	16	15	14	13	12	11	10	9	8	7	6	5	4	3	2	1
Drug	Dose															
tri-iodothyronine (T$_3$) (20 µg.tablet^{-1}.d^{-1}) (oral)											2	3	4	2	3	4
tetra-iodothyronine (T$_4$) (25 µg.tablet^{-1}.d^{-1}) (oral)											4	6	8	4	6	8
ephedrine (oral) (30 mg.tablet^{-1}.d^{-1})							3	3	6	6	8	8	8	8	8	8

IM = Intramuscular (parenteral) administration;
d^{-1} = daily dose; week^{-1} = weekly dose.

The stacking of AAS preparations has been the most commonly used method by bodybuilders. This concept of using smaller doses of different drugs with similar actions has been well established in the medical field. The overall idea has been to minimise the potential side effects and maximise the effectiveness of the regimes. Taking smaller dosages of multiple drugs may reduce the chance of liver abnormalities when compared to huge dosages of a single drug.

There is also evidence to suggest that there may be an increased liver tolerance to a smaller dose of multiple drugs compared to a large dose of a single anabolic agent. This increased tolerance would allow the liver to increase its degradation of one particular drug, in much lower concentrations. This may also facilitate the administration of multiple anabolic agents for longer periods, minimising the plateauing effect (Taylor, 1982). Bodybuilders are known to misuse enormous dosages of AAS, which have contributed to dyslipoproteinaemia, hyperhomocysteinaemia and premature death (Graham et al., 2006). In tables 2 and 3 are examples of the illegal cocktails and current dosages which are being promoted, equating to excessive weekly doses of thousands of milligrammes.

DRUG TESTING

Since AAS are often metabolised extensively, with little parent steroid being excreted into the urine, identification of metabolites for drug monitoring purposes is required. For many steroids there is more than one diagnostic metabolite. In man, the chemical synthesis of the major metabolites and their gas chromatography (GC) retention times change according to the GC/mass spectography (MS) method used, so the most important parameter described, is the mass spectrum of the metabolites [52].

In 1969, the first application of radioimmunoassay (RIA) for the measurement of steroids in biological fluids was published [53]. At that time there were 14 licensed orally active AAS. These steroids have a common 17 α-alkyl substituent (12 with a 17 α-methyl group and two with a 17 α-ethyl group). The method of detection used was to raise immunoglobulins that could target these two alkyl functions [54] Any presumptive positive samples could then be analysed by gas chromatography-mass spectrometry (GC/MS) for confirmatory identification [55]. A trial test targeting the orally active alkylated steroids was introduced at the Commonwealth Games in New Zealand in February 1974. Nine of 55 samples failed the immunoassay screen and seven samples confirmed positive by GC/MS. In April 1974, the IOC Medical Commission introduced AAS as a banned class of compounds in the Anti-Doping Code. In 1979 RIA screens were developed to detect the presence of nandrolone in urine, this AAS being manufactured for intramuscular injection [56]. Subsequently RIAs were developed for nandrolone metabolites [57]. In the 1980's improvements in the MS allowed IOC-accredited laboratories to develop specific and comprehensive screens able to detect ≤ 1ug/L of an AAS and its metabolite in urine [58]. The advantages that GC/MS screen provided, resulted in the replacement of RIA as the accepted method.

This testing brought about a change in the attitude of researchers regarding the use of anabolic agents. There was a shift in emphasis from defining the actions of anabolic steroids in the body, to sophisticated methods of detection.

Since 1969, the analysis techniques have grown to include every class of anabolic steroid used by athletes. Methods were originally proposed for determination of testosterone/gonadotrophin ratio in an attempt to discourage the use of exogenous testosterone by athletes [59] AAS detection has always been problematic. AAS are abused by athletes during training and are usually not taken during the actual competitive period, in an attempt to avoid detection. Since oral preparations are cleared from the body between 2-14 days following withdrawal, and water-soluble "injectables" after 4 weeks, it is possible to use these agents during periods of intensive training and test negative for the active metabolite. According to the 2009 WADA statistics [60], AAS are still the most frequent adverse analytical findings in- and out-of-competition.

Being aware of the pharmacokinetics of a wide variety of preparations, knowledge of a drug's half-life and detection methods has made it possible for some athletes to "pass the test". When attempts were made to arrest the abuse of AAS, athletes started to use the hormone testosterone, on the assumption that a test could not be produced to detect a substance that the body produces naturally.

The combination of the GC/MS and the Gas chromatography/combustion/ isotope-ratio mass spectrometry (GC/C/IRMS) analysis of urinary steroids was introduced to doping control in 1994 [61].

Synthesized steroids are normally made from Dioscorea species or soya. These are C3-plants, which are depleted in 13C in contrast to C4-plants. In consequence, synthesized steroids and their metabolites are also depleted in 13C in contrast to endogenous steroids since endogenous steroids derive from the diet, which is usually a mixture of C3-plants and C4-plants. 13C/12C-ratios of NA, androsterone and etiocholanolone measured by GC/C/IRMS offers a powerful tool to discriminate between the natural and synthetic origin of the urinary steroid 19-norandrosterone (NA). Due to the sensitivity of the instrument, this technology is more used by the laboratory for the testosterone detection than for the detection of nandrolone metabolites. NA is the most abundant metabolite of the synthetic anabolic steroid 19-nortestosterone and related prohormones [62].

In 1982, the IOC test for detection of testosterone administration was based on the GC/MS determination of the urinary ratio of testosterone (T) to its 17 α-epimer, epitestosterone (E), following glucuronide hydrolysis, commonly referred to as T/E ratio [63]. The T/E decision limit was derived empirically from an observed distribution of measurements in specimens collected from a large number of individuals. In healthy men and women, the T/E ratio is approximately 1. Supraphysiological doses of administered testosterone cause an increase in the ratio as a result of increased excretion of testosterone. The T/E ratio may be augmented as a consequence of dose-dependent inhibition of testicular steroidogenesis. When supraphysiological doses of testosterone are taken, suppression of LH secretion decreases urinary epitestosterone glucuronide. Intramuscular administration of 200 mg of testosterone enanthate weekly for 16 weeks decreases urinary E to < 10% of pre-administration values [64].

World Anti Doping Association (WADA) Medical Code stipulates that if a ratio of T/E is greater than 4, it is mandatory that the relevant medical authority conducts an investigation before the sample is declared positive. Because of natural variation of T/E ratios, if GC-IRMS does not verify exogenous administration, no further analysis is required [60;65]. Urine is the preferred biological fluid for detection of drugs of abuse. Independent sampling officers in the UK must witness a urine sample being delivered into a collection vessel. The sample kits and the chain-of-custody documentation must be able to withstand legal challenges. The athlete must pass urine equally into two coded glass bottles, each assigned a unique code. The samples are designated 'A-sample' approximately 70 mL and 'B-sample' approximately 30 mL for confirmatory analysis. The bottles are sealed using tamper-proof lids and then sent to the laboratory within a sealed shipping container. The independent sampling officer is also required to measure the pH and specific gravity of the urine.

When samples reach the laboratory, the A-sample seal is broken and the urine analysed. If the A-sample fails a drug test, the B-sample seal is broken at a later date and the analysis repeated. The failed drug sample athlete or sports person has the option to witness this procedure with an independent scientific expert and a legally qualified representative. Urine specimens are collected from individuals at multiple locations within a country, therefore transport difficulties may lead to delays of several days. Storage of samples in IOC-accredited laboratories is at $+4\ °C$ or $-20\ °C$. In the UK, samples are stored at $-20\ °C$. AAS are not thermally labile, but there has been concern about the possibility of microbial production of testosterone at temperatures that can lead to urine degradation causing positive urinary results [66]. Markers of degradation include a pH > 8.3 and/or a high level of 5α-androstenedione and free steroids that were originally glucuronidated (androsterone; etiocholanolone). In 2002, it was demonstrated that T can be elevated by inoculation of urine with Candida Albicans, but not at a level that would test positive [67]. However, such research has led to reversals of previous doping convictions.

The existing detection arrangements are proving successful. Offenders are being deterred, and prosecuted. But there is still potential for evasion, by cycling AAS out of season and evading doping tests. Principles are continuously being enhanced and incorporated into a more sophisticated drug testing regime.

A more recent determinant of long-term intermittent doping, is the provision of an athlete biological passport, which will demonstrate serial blood and urine analyses. Approximately 3,300 more samples were analysed in 2009 than in 2008, by WADA. (a total of 277,928 samples were analysed in 2009.) There was an increase in the number of Adverse Analytical Findings and Atypical Findings from 5,061 (2008) to 5,610 (2009).There was a slight increase in the global percentage of findings (which include Adverse

Analytical Findings and Atypical Findings) from 1.84% (2008) to 2.02% (2009) [65].

WADA's primary goal is to establish a level playing field for athletes worldwide by ensuring that all athletes are subjected to the same anti-doping protocols. Rather than using random selection to pick all athletes to be tested, WADA has adopted a scientific approach and selects a significant proportion of athletes based on several key factors, including their recent performance, history of doping, and vulnerability to the temptation to take performance-enhancing substances. WADA does not have its own sample collection personnel, but works in partnership with selected sample collection authorities worldwide. Samples are always sent to WADA-accredited laboratories. The 2009 adverse analytical findings (AAF) and atypical findings (AF) should not be confused with adjudicated or sanctioned anti-doping rules violations (ADRVs) for several reasons. First, these figures may contain findings that underwent the therapeutic use exemption (TUE) approval process. In addition, some AAFs and AFs may correspond to multiple findings on the same athlete or measurements performed on the same athlete, such as in cases of longitudinal studies in testosterone (i.e., tracking the testosterone level of one athlete over a period of time).

In 2005, WADA began the roll out of anti-doping administration and management system (ADAMS), a Web-based database management tool for athletes and anti-doping organizations. ADAMS is a platform for results management, administration of TUEs, athlete whereabouts information, and test distribution planning. With the full adoption of ADAMS by stakeholders, the sporting community will have a transparent means for tracking results, from collection to sanction, while respecting confidentiality. In addition, complete analysis of data will be available, including linking Adverse Analytical Findings to TUEs and sanctioned cases. In the interim, International Federations (IFs) and National Anti-Doping Organizations (NADOs), as part of their Code responsibilities, are obliged to report their testing statistics directly to WADA at least annually; also as required by the Code, WADA publicly reports data received from IFs and NADOs.

CONCLUSION

Implementing testing procedures is difficult since few amateur sporting bodies have the financial resources available to make the programmes effective. Amateur sport is the breeding ground for professional sport. Testing has not extended into competitive bodybuilding, which has remained immune, in contrast to sports like athletics, in which the sports council has spent significant sums on testing programmes. Past surveys identifying levels of AAS abuse may have been skewed by the concentration on hard-core gymnasia. However, with the prosecution of high profile athletes and the administration of lighter sentences to obtain co-operation in identifying sources of drug use and drug users, the extent is only just becoming apparent.

The consensus of opinion of scientific colleagues is there is widespread cheating with many authorities burying their heads in the sand and that WADA are fighting an unwinnable war [68]. A controversial solution which has been called for is the introduction of a chemical level playing field. An Olympic games where athletes use ergogenic aids freely, under medical supervision, in a controlled environment, which more importantly would contribute to scientific research and minimise the risks to the athletes themselves [69].

REFERENCES

[1]   David, KG; Dingemanse, E; Freud, J; Laqueur, E. On crystalline male hormones from testicles(testosterone) effective as from urine or from cholesterol. *Hoppe Seylers Z Physiol Chem.*, 1935 233, 281.

[2]   Butenandt, A; Hanisch, G. About Testosterone. Conversion of Dehydro-androsterone into androstendiol and testosterone; a way for the structure assignment of testosterone from cholestrol. *Hoppe Seylers Z Physiol Chem.*, 1935a 237, 89.

[3]   Butenandt, A; Hanisch, G. The conversion of dehydroandrosterone into androstenol-(17)-one-3 (testosterone); a method for the production of testosterone from cholesterol. *Chemische Berichte*, 1935b 68, 1859–1862.

[4]   Ruzicka, L; Wettstein, A. The crystalline production of the testicle hormone, testosterone (Androsten-3-ol-17-ol]. *Helvetica Chimica Acta*, 1935 18, 1264–1275.

[5]   Kenyon, AT; Knowlton, K; Sandiford, I; Koch, FC; Lotwin,G. (1940). A comparative study of the metabolic effects of testosterone propionate in normal men and women and in eunuchoidism. *Endocrinology*, 1940 26, 26–45.

[6]   Shahidi, NT. A review of the chemistry, biological action, and clinical applications of anabolic-androgenic steroids. *Clin. Ther.*, 2001 23, 1355-1390.

[7]   Wilson, JD; Leihy, MW; Shaw, G; Renfree, MB. Androgen physiology: unsolved problems at the millennium. *Mol. Cell Endocrinol.*, 2002 198, 1-5.

[8]   Janne, OA; Palvimo, JJ; Kallio, P; Mehto, M. Androgen receptor and Mechanism of androgen action. *Ann. Med.*, 1993 25, 83-89.

[9]   Deslypere, JP; Young, M; Wilson, JD; McPhaul, MJ. Testosterone and 5 alpha-dihydrotestosterone interact differently with the androgen receptor to enhance transcription of the MMTV-CAT reporter gene. *Mol. Cell Endocrinol.*, 1992 88, 15-22.

[10] Kroon, FJ; Munday, PL; Westcott, DA; Hobbs, JP; Liley, NR. Aromatase pathway mediates sex change in each direction. *Proc. Biol. Sci.*, 2005 272, 1399-1405.

[11] Bhasin, S; Storer, TW; Berman, N; Callegari, C; Clevenger, B; Phillips, J; Bunnell, TJ; Tricker, R; Shirazi, A; Casaburi, R. The effects of supraphysiologic doses of testosterone on muscle size and strength in normal men. *N. Engl. J. Med.*, 1996 335, 1-7.

[12] Pope, H; Phillips, K; Olivardia, R. The Adonis Complex- The secret crisis of male body obsession. *New York: The Free Press*, 2000 11.

[13] Brower, KJ. (2002). Anabolic steroid abuse and dependence. *Curr. Psychiatry. Rep.*, 2002 4, 377-387.

[14] Graham, MR; Baker, JS; Davies, B. "Steroid" and prescription medicine abuse in the health and fitness community; a regional study. *Eur. J. Intern. Med.*, 2006a 17, 479-484.

[15] Voy, R. Drugs, Sport and Politics. *Leisure press.* Champaign, Illinois, 1991.

[16] Gold, J; Batterham, MJ; Rekers, H; Harms, MK; Geurts, TB; Helmyr, PM; Silva de Mendonça, J; Falleiros, Carvalho, LH; Panos, G; Pinchera, A; Aiuti, F; Lee, C; Horban, A; Gatell, J; Phanuphak, P; Prasithsirikul, W; Gazzard, B; Bloch, M; Danner, SA. Effects of nandrolone decanoate compared with placebo or testosterone on HIV-associated wasting. *HIV Med.*, 2006 7, 146-155.

[17] Cramer, RJ. Anabolic steroids are easily purchased without a prescription and present significant challenges to law enforcement officials. *United States Government Accountability Office.* 2005 Available at http://www.gao.gov/new.items/d06243r.pdf. Accessed 17 July 2011.

[18] Hermansson, G. Doping trade: business for the big ones. In: Play the Game, 2002 http://www.anasci.org/vB/anabolic-steroid-articles/8440-interesting-article-swedish-police.html. Accessed 17 July 2011.

[19] Graham, MR; Ryan, P; Baker, JS; Davies, B; Thomas, NE; Cooper, SM; Evans, P; Easmon, S; Walker, CJ; Cowan, D; Kicman, AT. (2009). Counterfeiting in performance- and image *Drug Test. Anal.*, 2009 1, 135-1342.

[20] Grace, FM; Baker, JS; Davies, B. Anabolic Androgenic Steroid (AAS) Use in Recreational Gym Users- A regional sample of the Mid-Glamorgan area. *J. Substance Use*, 2001 12, 145-153.

[21] Parkinson, AB; Evans, NA. Anabolic androgenic steroids: a survey of 500 users. *Med. Sci. Sports Exerc.*, 2006 38, 644-651.

[22] Graham, MR; Grace, FM; Boobier, W; Hullin, D; Kicman, A; Cowan, D; Davies, B; Baker, JS. Homocysteine induced cardiovascular events: a consequence of long term anabolic-androgenic steroid (AAS) abuse. *Br. J. Sports Med.*, 2006b 40, 644-648.

[23] Graham, MR; Davies, B; Grace, FM; Kicman, A; Baker, JS. Anabolic steroid use: patterns of use and detection *Sports Med.*, 2008 38, 505-525.

[24] Mooradian, AD; Morley, JE; Korenman, SG. (1987). Biological actions of androgens. *Endocr. Rev.*, 1987 8, 1-28.

[25] Devoto, CE; Madariaga, AM; Lioi, CX; Mardones, N. Influence of size and duration of gynecomastia on its response to treatment with tamoxifen. *Rev. Med. Chil.*, 2007 135, 1558-1565.

[26] Buccilli, TA, Jr; Hall, HR; Solmen, JD. Sterile abscess formation following a corticosteroid injection for the treatment of plantar fasciitis. *J Foot Ankle Surg.*, 2005 44, 466-468.

[27] Rich, JD; Dickinson, BP; Flanigan, TP; Valone SE. Abscesses related to anabolic-androgenic steroid injection. *Med. Sci. Sports Exerc.*, 1999 31, 207-09.

[28] Maropis, C; Yesalis, CE. Intramuscular abscess: another anabolic steroid danger. *Physician Sportsmed.,* 1994 22, 105-10.

[29] Marquis, CP; Maffulli, N. Anabolic steroid related abscess-A risk worth taking? *Injury Extra*, 2006 12, 451-454.

[30] Plaus, WJ; Hermann, G. The surgical management of superficial infections caused by atypical mycobacteria. *Surgery,* 1991 110, 99-105.

[31] Nemechek, PM. Anabolic steroid users: another potential risk group for HIV infection. *NEJM,* 1991 325, 357.

[32] Vlahov, D; Normand, J; Moses, LE. *Preventing HIV Transmission: the Role of Sterile Needles and Bleach.* National Research Council. *Washington, DC: National Academy Press*, 1995 170, 53-82.

[33] Dickinson, BP; Rich JD; Flanigan, TP. Anabolic steroid injectors and needle exchange programs in the United States: 1996. *North American Syringe Exchange Network Conference.* San Diego, CA, 1997 April 23-26.

[34] McCreaddie, M; Lyons, I; Horsburgh, D; Miller, M; Frew, J. The isolating and insulating effects of hepatitis *Gastroenterol Nurs.*, 2011 34, 49-59.

[35] Aceijas, C; Rhodes, T. Global estimates of prevalence of HCV infection among injecting drug users. *Int. J. Drug Policy*, 2007 18, 352-358.

[36] Chak, E; Talal, AH; Sherman, KE; Schiff, ER; Saab, S. Hepatitis C virus infection *Liver Int.*, 2011 doi:10.1111/j.1478-3231.2011.02494. Epub ahead of print.

[37] Turner, K; Hutchinson, S; Vickerman, P; Hope, V; Craine, N; Palmateer, N; May, M; Taylor, A; De Angelis, D; Cameron, S; Parry, J; Lyons, M; Goldberg, D; Allen, E; Hickman, M. The impact of needle and syringe provision and opiate substitution *Addiction*, 2011 doi: 10.1111/j.1360-0443.2011.03515. Epub ahead of print.

[38] Waddington, I. Doping In Sport: Some Issues for Medical Practitioners. *Physical Education and Sport*, 2001 1, 51 – 59.

[39] Franke, WW; Berendonk, B. Hormonal doping and androgeniization of athletes: a secret program of the German Democratic Republic Goverment. *Clin Chem.*, 1997 43, 1262-1279.

[40] Fair, JD. Isometrics or Steroids? Exploring New Frontiers of Strength in the Early 1960s. *Journal of Sport History*, 1993 20, 1.

[41] Dubin, CL (The Honourable). Commission of Inquiry into the Use of Drugs and banned Practices Intended to increase Athletic Performance. Ottawa: *Canadian Government Publishing Centre.* 1990.

[42] Bamberger, M; Yaeger, D. Over the edge. *Sports Illustrated*, 1997 14, 62-70.

[43] Catlin, DH; Sekera, MH; Ahrens, BD; Starcevic B, Chang YC, Hatton CK. Tetrahydrogestrinone: discovery, synthesis, and detection in urine. Rapid Commun. *Mass Spectrom.*, 2004 18, 1245-1249.

[44] Mitchell, GJ. Report to the Commissioner of Baseball of an Independent Investigation into the Illegal Use of Steroids and Other Performance Enhancing Substances by Players in Major League Baseball. *DLA Piper US LLP.* 2007 1-409.

[45] Ferenchick, GS; Hirokawa, S; Mammen, EF; Schwartz, KA. Anabolic-androgenic steroid abuse in weight lifters: evidence for activation of the hemostatic system. *Am. J. Hematol.*, 1995 49, 282-288.

[46] Di Pasquale, MG. *Anabolic Steroid Side-Effects. Facts, Fiction and Treatment.* Edition. Ontario: MGD Press 1990.

[47] Cicardi, M; Bergamischini, L; Tucci, A; Agostoni, A; Tornaghi, G; Coggi, G; Colombi, R; Viale, G. Morphological evaluation of the liver in hereditary angioedema patients on long-term treatment with androgen derivatives. *J. Allergy Clin. Immunol.*, 1983 72, 294-298.

[48] Miyamoto, H; Yeh, S; Lardy, H; Messing, E; Chang, C. Delta 5-androstenediol is a natural hormone with androgenic activity in human prostate cancer cells. *Proc. Natl. Acad. Sci.* USA, 1998 95, 11083-11088.

[49] Van der Vies, J. Pharmacokinetics of anabolic steroids. *Wien Med. Wochenschr.*, 1993 143, 366-8.

[50] Hartgens, F; Rietjens, G; Keizer, HA; et al. Effects of androgenic-anabolic steroids on apolipoproteins and lipoprotein (a). *Br. J. Sports Med.*, 2004 38, 253-259.

[51] Taylor, WN. *Anabolic Steroids and the Athlete.* Mcfarland 1982.

[52] Schanzer, W; Donike, M. Metabolism of anabolic steroids in man: synthesis and use of reference substances for identification of anabolic steroid metabolites. *Anal. Chim. Acta.*, 1993 275, 23-48.

[53] Abraham, GE. Solid-phase radioimmunoassay of estradiol-17-β. *J. Clin. Endocrinol. Metab.*, 1969 29, 866-870.

[54] Brooks, RV; Firth, RG; Sumner, NA. Detection of anabolic steroids by radioimmunoassay. *Br. J. Sports Med.*, 1975 9, 89-92.

[55] Ward, RJ; Shackleton, CH; Lawson, AM. Gas chromatographic-mass spectrometric methods for the detection and identification of anabolic steroid drugs. *Br. J. Sports Med.*, 1975 9, 93-97.

[56] Brooks, RV; Jeremiah, G; Webb, WA; Wheeler, M. Detection of anabolic steroid administration to athletes. *J. Steroid Biochem.*, 1979 11, 913-917.

[57] Kicman, AT; Brooks, RV. Radioimmunoassay for Nandrolone metabolites. *J. Pharm. Biomed. Anal.*, 1988 6, 473-83.

[58] Catlin, DH; Kammerer, RC; Hatton, CK; Sekera, MH; Merdink, JL. Analytical chemistry at the Games of the XXIIIrd Olympiad in Los Angeles, 1984. *Clin. Chem.*, 1987 33, 319-27.

[59] Benjamin, IS. *The Case against Anabolic Steroids. Medicine Sport and the Law.* SDW Payne (Ed): Blackwell Scientific Publications; 1990.

[60] http://www.wada-ama.org/en/World-Anti-Doping-Program/Sports-and-Anti-Doping-Organizations/International-Standards/Prohibited-List/The-2011-Prohibited-List/

[61] Becchi, M; Aguilera, R; Farizon, Y; Flament, MM;, Casabianca, H; James P. Gas chromatography/combustion/isotope-ratio mass spectrometry analysis of urinary steroids to detect misuse of testosterone in sport. *Rapid Commun. Mass Spectrom.*, 1994 8, 304–308.

[62] Hebestreit, M; Flenker, U; Fussholler, G; Geyer, H; Güntner, U; Mareck, U; Piper, T; Thevis, M; Ayotte, C; Schänzer, W. Determination of the origin of urinary norandrosterone traces by gas chromatography combustion isotope ratio mass spectrometry. *Analyst.* 2006 131, 1021-6.

[63] Donike, M; Barwald, KR; Klosterman, K. Detection of exogenous testosterone. In: Heck H, Hollman W, Liesen H, et al., eds. Sport: *Leistung und Gesundheit, Kongressbd. Dtsch. Sportarztekongress.* Koln: Deutscher Artze-Verlag 1983 293-298.

[64] Anderson, RA; Wallace, AM; Kicman, AT; Wu, FC. Comparison between testosterone oenanthate-induced azoospermia and oligospermia in a male contraceptive study. IV. Suppression of endogenous testicular and adrenal androgens. *Hum. Reprod.*, 1997 12, 1657-1662.

[65] http://www.wada-ama.org/rtecontent/document/LABSTATS_2010.PDF.

[66] Bilton, RF. Microbial production of testosterone. *Lancet*, 1995 345, 1186-1187.

[67] Kicman, AT; Fallon, JK; Cowan, DA; Walker, C; Easmon, S; Mackintosh, D. Candida albicans can produce testosterone: impact on the T/E sports drug test. *Clin. Chem.*, 2002 10, 1799-801.

[68] Savulescu, J; Foddy, B; Clayton, M. Why we should allow performance-enhancing drugs in sport. *Br. J. Sports Med.*, 2004 38, 666-670.

[69] Kayser, B; Mauron, A; Miah, A. Viewpoint: Legalisation of performance-enhancing drugs. *Lancet*, 2005 1, 21.

[70] Kicman, AT; Gower, DB. Anabolic steroids in sport: biochemical, clinical and analytical perspectives. *Ann. Clin. Biochem.*, 2003 40, 321-356.

Sport and Exercise Science, Institute of Health, Medical Science and Society Science, Glyndwr University, Wrexham, Wales, United Kingdom, LL11 2AW.

In: Perspectives on Anabolic Androgenic ….   ISBN: 978-1-62081-243-3
Editors: F. Grace and J. S. Baker   © 2012 Nova Science Publishers, Inc.

Chapter 2

TESTOSTERONE AND MOLECULAR REGULATION OF SKELETAL MUSCLE

D. C. Hughes[1], N. Sculthorpe[1], A. P. Sharples[1] and M. P. Lewis[2,1,3]

[1]Muscle Cellular and Molecular Research Group, Institute of Sport and Physical Activity Research, University of Bedfordshire, UK
[2]Molecular and Cellular Physiology, Musculoskeletal Biology Research Group, School of Sport, Health and Exercise Science, Loughborough University, Loughborough, UK
[3]School of Life and Medical Sciences, University College London (UCL), UK

ABSTRACT

Androgen endocrine physiology is responsible for many processes in the body, from bone metabolism to skeletal muscle maintenance. Testosterone (T) is one of the most potent androgens produced, with decades of research highlighting its androgenic-anabolic effect on skeletal muscle growth. The research has been further driven through the emergence of pharmaceutical derivates (steroids) of T and their use in interventions for muscle wasting associated with disease and advancing age (sarcopenia). However, the molecular regulation of T and the influence it has on cellular processes in promoting muscle development, hypertrophy and satellite cell activation (proliferation, differentiation) remain poorly understood. The utilisation of human, animal models and cell culture have begun to suggest the molecular mechanisms by which T acts on skeletal muscle, yet often the results remain inconclusive. This review therefore highlights the most current research into the molecular mechanisms of T with suggested future direction. An emergent feature is the possible lack of biomimicity between monolayer cell culture models and the *in-vivo* environment. Bio-engineered skeletal muscle thus represents a physiological tool to bridge the gap by incorporating a native cell niche and extracellular environment that skeletal muscle has *in-vivo*. With future experimentation and by unravelling key cellular and molecular mechanisms of testosterone regulation there is the potential to harness the un-refutable power of this hormone in order to implement interventions for sarcopenia and muscle wasting diseases.

INTRODUCTION

Testosterone (17β-Hydroxyandrost-4-en-3-one: $C_{19}H_{28}O_2$) is a potent naturally occurring steroid hormone (androgen) produced from cholesterol. Within the body, testosterone (T) is responsible for regulating many physiological processes such as muscle maintenance, sexual and cognitive function, plasma lipids and bone metabolism [1, 2]. For decades, testosterone has been researched from the perspective of these physiological processes, with muscle growth, development and maintenance receiving predominant attention. Furthermore, such attention to muscle growth has been highlighted through the emergence of chemical and pharmaceutical derivates of T called Androgenic-Anabolic Steroids (AAS) [2, 3]. The molecular regulation of T and its pharmaceutical derivatives remain poorly understood. Recent research however, has begun to delve into these mechanisms alongside the emergence of new cellular and molecular technologies. This chapter will summarise the current research underpinning the action of molecular regulation by T and its role in growth in skeletal muscle and highlight future directions.

The aging process correlates with a gradual decline in the production of testosterone and a subsequent reduction in serum T levels [4]. In healthy young men, serum T levels range from 400-1000 ng/dl [5, 6] whereas for elderly men, serum testosterone levels range from 150-550 ng/dl [16]. Any serum T levels below this range for elderly men are defined as hypogonadism [4]. Declining serum levels highlight the effects that T may have on peripheral tissues where sarcopenia and osteoporosis have been previously associated with the reduced levels [4, 7]. Testosterone administration has been utilised as a treatment for such conditions, and more importantly the development of T derivatives and selective androgen receptor modulators (SARMs) has provided a more specific target of action within the treatment of tissues [4,8]. However, due to its clinical importance it is fundamentally important to first understand the mechanisms and signalling pathways that T and androgens activate, to reduce the risk of cross talk with other signalling pathways and thus potential side effects that could be incurred with such pharmaceutical treatments (discussed below).

Testosterone Production *in-vivo*

Testosterone is produced predominately in the leydig cells located in the testes of males, with a small amount being additionally secreted from the adrenal cortex and ovaries in females. The nature of the hormone prevents it from being stored in the cells that produce it and thus on production, it is immediately released from the cells. The signalling for the production of T within the gonads is through the hypothalamic-pituitary-gonadal-axis (Figure 1.) [9,10]. The signal originates in the hypothalamus by innervations of the Central Nervous System (CNS) which leads to specialized neurons secreting gonadotropin-releasing hormone (GnRH). GnRH is then transported from the hypothalamus to the anterior pituitary gland and subsequently to the pituitary target cells, via the hypothalamic-hypophysical portal vein. At this location, GnRH activates the production and release of lutenizing hormone (LH) and follicle-stimulating hormone (FSH) from the gonadotropes, with both hormones consequently circulating to the gonads (Figure 1.).

Lutenizing hormone is responsible for testosterone production in the leydig cells in men and the theca calls in women. This production is brought about by LH binding to a G-protein coupled membrane receptor [11, 12]. Furthermore, the binding process initiates a rate-limiting step in testosterone production by way of cyclic adenosine monophosphate dependant protein kinase (protein kinase A) stimulation [11, 12]. On the other hand, in terms of variations between men and women, FSH appears to have no direct effect on testosterone stimulation in men but stimulates production of pregrendone in women. Pregnenolone is further processed into testosterone upon leaving the granuolsa cells. Another role of FSH, which appears in both men and women, is the stimulation of steroid binding proteins in the liver. These proteins (primary being sex-hormone binding globulin) are especially important for the T produced to be circulated within the body, due to testosterone's hydrophobic nature and thus are not readily dissolved within the blood [10].

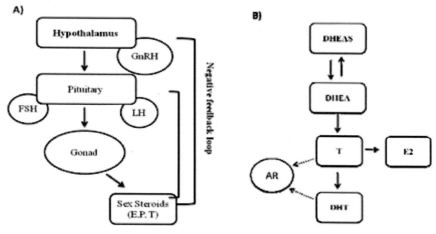

(Adapted from Vandenput and Ohlsson [15]; Wierman [16]).

Figure 1. Testosterone is produced through the signalling events of the Hypothalamus-pituitary-gondal axis (A) and alternatively synthesised in target tissues via androgen metabolism (B). E, estrogen; P, progesterone; T, testosterone; E2, estradiol; AR, androgen receptor; DHEA, dehydroepiandrosterone; DHEAS, dehydroepiandrosterone sulphate.

Although this cascade of signalling events is the predominant source for T and androgen production, about 30 to 50% of androgens are further produced in peripheral tissues [13, 14].

Peripheral Tissue Expression

Androgen production in peripheral tissue, such as bone and skeletal muscle, is synthesized locally from the sex steroid precursor's dehydroepiandrosterone (DHEA) and DHEA sulphate (Figure 1.) [15, 17]. The transformation of both steroid precursors involves steroidogenic enzymes to produce T and various other androgens (Figure 1.). Of these steroidgenic enzymes, 5-α reductase is critical in converting T to dihydrotestosterone (DHT) [14, 15]. In both male and female rats, a single bout of exercise has been show to increase all of these metabolites (DHEA, DHEAS, T, DHT and 5-α reductase type 1 isoenzyme) and thus the activation of local bioactive androgen metabolism [18]. Ultimately, the conversion creates a more potent androgen in DHT and is more readily available within the tissue compared to testosterone [19]. A characteristic for DHT being more potent is the higher binding affinity to the androgen receptor within the cells [19]. Although within skeletal muscle, DHT levels are considerably low compared to T due to the low levels of 5-α reductase [20].

In bone tissue, bio available testosterone is converted to estradiol through aromatization (Figure 1.), with estradiol being observed to be important for regulation of bone loss and bone metabolism [15, 23, 24]. Therefore, a reduced level with increasing age or even a testosterone/estradiol deficiency within individuals has been associated with rapid bone loss, in turn impacting on bone mineral content and density, leading to a more prevalent incidence of osteoporosis in elderly men and women [25]. Estradiol has repeatedly been associated as the main predictor of bone morphology, with T frequently showing no association in bone structural parameters. Testosterones role within bone remodelling is believed to be primarily centred on its availability for conversion to estradiol [26]. Although, a recent study by Ward et al. [26] suggests that bio-available T may influence bone health through its effect on skeletal muscle mass reducing mechanical load inducing bone remodelling. For a more detailed review on sex steroid metabolism and influences on bone, refer to Vandenput and Ohlsson [15] or Callewaert, Boonen and Vanderschueren [27]. For the purpose of this review chapter, the main focus will be the molecular aspects of testosterone signalling in skeletal muscle cells and the current understanding of T's molecular role within skeletal muscle maintenance, growth and development.

TESTOSTERONE AND SKELETAL MUSCLE

Testosterone elicits an anabolic effect on skeletal muscle via increases in protein synthesis, decreases in protein degradation and the reutilization of amino acids [28-30]. These adaptations culminate in a hypertrophic (increased size via increased protein synthesis) response occurring in skeletal muscle. Indeed, a dose dependant increase in the size of skeletal muscle, shown by increases in cross sectional area (CSA), is observed following administration of testosterone enanthate at doses of 25-600mg [1, 31, 32]. Another form of growth within skeletal muscle, besides hypertrophy, is muscle cell hyperplasia. Skeletal muscle fibre number is set at gestation (*in-utero*) due to mature fibres that are unable to divide (i.e. terminally differentiated or post mitotic). Skeletal muscle's change in size occurs as a result of a specialised cell type (the satellite cell) that resides underneath the basal lamina. These cells can undergo hyperplasia (cell division/ mitosis) and fuse to the existing fibres to increase size or repair damage from trauma, injury or exercise. Testosterone has been shown to increase satellite cell number and increase activation and fusion of these cells indicated by an increase in myonuclear incorporation in skeletal muscle *in-vivo* following testosterone administration (100-600mg) [20,33]. The analysis of skeletal muscle morphology in power lifters demonstrates significant positive correlations between the number of myonuclei per area and fibre area size [34]. Indeed, with the use of androgenic-anabolic steroids, muscle hypertrophy adaptations in power lifter users are amplified compared to non-users [34]. Despite these intriguing physiological observations, the molecular mechanisms by which testosterone initiates anabolic processes for a hypertrophic response remain poorly understood.

To investigate androgen signalling, various experimental approaches have been utilised. Commonly, the administration of exogenous T [35] is implemented, employed in either an *in-vivo* or *in-vitro* model. Alternatively the suppression of endogenous testosterone within *in-vivo* models, via injections (goserelin), are performed [36]. Other molecular techniques have enabled research to gain an insight into T's mechanisms using androgen receptor antagonists [37, 38] and transgenic or knock out animal models [39, 40]. Another approach within *in-vivo* studies is the elevation in endogenous serum T levels (up to $38nmol.L^{-1}$ (1100ng/dl)) through resistance training [41]. This response is commonly elicited through a high volume and high intensity program [10, 41]. Human muscle biopsies can be taken pre and post resistance training to enhance our understanding of molecular events associated with this specific stimulus and the role of T. However, due to ethical considerations and difficult sampling and processing of biopsies, this particular approach has been relatively unavailable in human studies. Therefore, animal and *in-vitro* models currently allow for the most in depth investigation of the molecular targets involved in androgen signalling, with the identification of potential target pathways to be triggered through a T stimulus. Below are some of the mechanisms indicated by these models.

DIRECT PATHWAY (TESTOSTERONE-AR COMPLEX)

Androgens interact with muscle tissue via the androgen receptor (AR), a member of the steroid receptor superfamily and nuclear transcription factors [20, 42]. The AR is detectable within hormone-sensitive cells e.g. bone and muscle cells [43]. Within target cells, un-ligand bound AR is located in the cytoplasmic compartment of the cell, in the form of a multi-complex protein consisting of heat shock proteins and immunophilins (Figure 2.) [19, 44]. Once testosterone is bound to AR, a conformational change occurs leading to AR dissociating from its multi-protein complex and recruiting co-activators such as importin-α, androgen receptor-associated protein-70 (ARA70) and filamin-α, enabling the ligand-bound AR to translocate to the nucleus (Figure 2.) [19, 45]. In the nucleus, AR acts as a transcription factor for specific target genes such as insulin-like growth factor I, MyoD, myosin heavy chains [43] and thus interacts with androgen responsive elements (ARE) within the genome [28]. Therefore, AR have been proposed to mediate an array of functions within skeletal muscle cells such as proliferation, differentiation into myotubes, and control apoptosis within skeletal muscle cells [19].

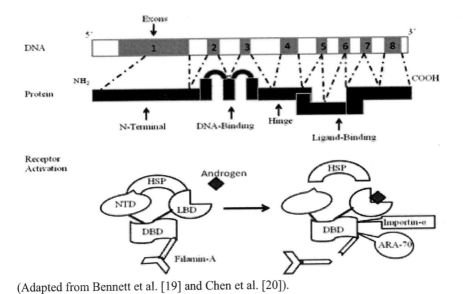

(Adapted from Bennett et al. [19] and Chen et al. [20]).

Figure 2. Overview of the human androgen receptor gene, protein and the conformational change once bound to an androgen. The gene consists of 8 exons which code for a functional protein (approx. 920 amino acids) with four domains. Exon 1 encodes for the N-terminal transactivation domain (NTD); Exon 2-3 encodes the DNA-binding domain (DBD); Exon 4 encodes the small hinge region, finally exons 5-8 encode for the C-terminal ligand-binding domain (LBD). The LBD represent the domain where androgens bind to the receptor protein, resulting in the release of heat shock proteins (HSP) and immunophilins plus the recruitment of co-activators, ARA70 and filamin-α, thus enabling translocation to the nucleus.

Satellite cells (discussed above) within skeletal muscle provide the predominant location for AR expression and thus androgens can act directly through these cells [20, 46, 47]. Satellite cells once activated are termed myoblasts and can proliferate, enter differentiation or even return to quiescence (Figure 3.) [20, 48, 49].

In addition, as mentioned satellite cells provide a major source for the addition of new myonuclei within the skeletal muscle [42] and thus the myonuclei addition increases the focal points for AR expression as well as helping maintain nuclear-to-cytoplasmic balance [50]. In terms of muscle hypertrophy, the differentiation/fusion of cells into the existing fibres allows for a further increase in size (Figure 3.). Plus the addition of more satellite cells, as previously mentioned, leading to an increased in myonuclei would aid in the availability of androgen receptors to interact with testosterone more readily [5]. The availability of the androgen receptor and testosterone levels is highlighted by gender differences, as males produce ten times more testosterone and equally have a higher AR protein content than in females [51].

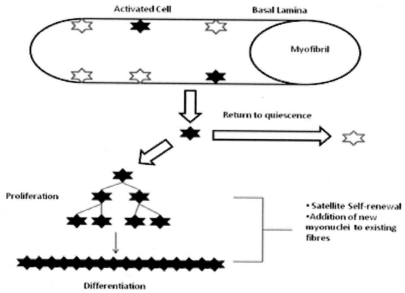

(Adapted from Kadi et al. [48]).

Figure 3. Location of the Satellite cell and its involvement in muscle fibre modeling.

In mediating T's effects, the increase (up-regulation) or decrease (down-regulation) in AR expression is an important consideration [51, 52]. Commonly with resistance exercise, where acute elevations in testosterone levels are observed, there is an initial stabilisation of the AR, followed by a down-regulation (1hr post exercise) [52] before finally an up-regulation (3hr post exercise [41]).

This type of phase response is further highlighted by Ferrando et al. [35] where the (6 months) administration of exogenous T produced a significant increase in AR protein expression after 1 month, yet after 6 months of administration, AR protein expression levels returned to near baseline values. Additionally, in females, this phase response occurs more quickly than in males [51].

The phase response or paradigm was suggested to be the result of a steady-state adaptation with the administration of T. Interestingly though, Insulin-Like Growth Factor I (IGF-I) protein expression, remained elevated for the same time frame after exogenous T administration.

Thus, the question is, does T's interaction revolve predominately around the AR or an indirect pathway, for which in the *in-vivo* environment, the administration of T may be more beneficial to patients in a cycling pattern [35]?

Two more recent *in-vivo* studies investigated the role of androgen receptor expression by suppressing endogenous T (by injecting goserelin) [36] or applying a resistance training stimulus to elevate endogenous T [28]. Through the implementation of a 21 week resistance training program (60-90% of 1 RM, 5-12 reps per set, 5 sets total), Athtianen et al. [28] observed no statistically significant changes in AR mRNA expression and AR protein content between young and old training groups.

However, when individual changes within groups were further analysed, significant relationships were observed in AR protein concentrations and training-induced changes (1 repetition maximum, fibre CSA) within the skeletal muscle i.e. increased AR protein concentration with increase in fibre CSA. Thus, AR protein concentrations may have a role within changes in training muscular adaptations.

Contrary to this, Korvning et al [36] suppressed testosterone which limited the increase in muscle strength being observed post-strength training but more importantly endogenous testosterone did not appear to be involved in the regulation of AR mRNA expression as similar expression was observed in suppressed vs. placebo groups. Indeed, recent research has suggested that testosterone may influence on skeletal muscle growth via a different pathway to AR interaction [43, 52, 53].

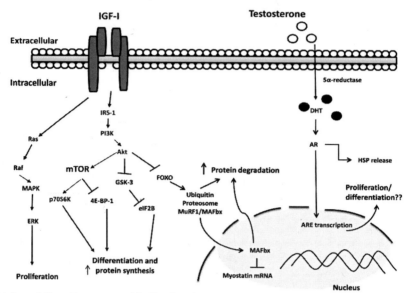

(Adapted from Bennett et al [19]; Sharples and Stewart [55]).

Figure 4. Two potential pathways testosterone may use to interact with skeletal muscle cells. Testosterone can act directly via the AR pathway (right side) or indirectly through the IGF-I signalling pathway (left side). Akt, protein kinase B; AR, Androgen receptor; ARE, Androgen response elements; DHT, dihydrotestosterone; ERK, extracellular signal-regulated kinase; eiF2B, the guanine nucleotide-exchange factor for eukaryotic initiation factor 2; 4E-BPP-1, eukaryotic translation initiation factor 4E binding protein 1; FOXO, forkhead homebox type O; GSK-3, Glycogen Synthase Kinase-3; HSP, Heat shock proteins; IGF-I, insulin-like growth factor-I; IRS-1, insulin receptor substrate-1; MAFbx, Muscle atrophy f-box; MAPK, mitogen activated protein kinase; mTOR, mammalian target of rapamycin; MuRF1, muscle RING-finger protein-1; P70S6K, P70S6 Kinase- a serine/threonine kinase (phosphorylation of S6 induces protein synthesis at the ribosome); Ras, Ras Protein; Raf, MAP Kinase Kinase Kinase (MAP3K).

INDIRECT PATHWAYS

Role of IGF-I and Its Downstream Pathways

IGF-I regulates several biochemical pathways (Figure 4.), involved in protein synthesis within skeletal muscle cells [56. 57]. The downstream pathways of Pi3K/Akt/mTOR play a fundamental role in myotube hypertrophy (Figure 4.) [57], with recent evidence that mTOR can be also activated independently of

IGF-I through mechanical stimulation and amino acid supplementation [58, 59]. The binding of IGF-I to its receptor, activates a cascade of signalling, initiated with the activation of Pi3K. The release of a phosphate group by Pi3K allows for the phosphorylation and activation of Akt. Once at this step in the pathway, Akt mediates the phosphorlaytion of mTOR. Through mTOR, protein synthesis is promoted through mitigating eukaryotic initiation factor 4E– binding protein 1 (4E-BP1)-mediated inhibition of eukaryotic initiation factor 4E (eIF-4E) [56, 57]. Supplementary to mTOR promoting protein synthesis through eIF-4E, the activation of mTOR further promotes protein synthesis via the phosporylation of p70S6k and subsequent S6K downstream target [56]. Another downstream target, GSk-3β is a substrate of Akt and thus once Akt is phosphorylated, GSk-3β becomes phosporylated and inhibited. This inhibition of GSk-3β in turn activates eukaryotic translation factor eIF-2B leading to further increases in protein synthesis (Figure 4.).There is evidence that testosterone mediates its androgenic effects through Insulin-like growth factor (IGF-I) and it's associated downstream signaling [60]. For example, with a T deficiency, a reduced level of IGF-I in humans has been observed which may suggest an activation/synergistic behaviour by testosterone on IGF-I [31, 56]. The suggested synergistic behaviour is further supported through T supplementation, where the addition of exogenous androgens is accompanied by an increase in IGF-I protein and mRNA expression [39, 60, 61]. Furthermore, IGF- I and its splice variants, IGF-IEa and MGF, stimulate both satellite cell proliferation and differentiation with a unique temporal expression following resistance exercise [62-64]. There is emerging evidence within skeletal muscle cells for IGF-I activation of the AR through a ligand-independent mechanism [65-67].

The androgen receptor is considered a ligand dependant receptor, yet recent research by Kim and Lee [66, 67] suggests that total AR, AR phosphorylation and increases in AR mRNA expression can be induced through the addition of endogenous IGF-I in C2C12 skeletal muscle cells. These nvestigators observed (through immunocytochemistry fluourescence staining) an increase in AR DNA binding activity in murine skeletal muscle cells (C2C12) in a time-dependant manner after being treated with IGF-I.. Therefore, in the presence of IGF-I, it was observed that AR localisation in the nucleus increased along with binding to ARE, in the absence of ligand. A follow up study by Kim and Lee [67] addressed the MAPK pathway (discussed in more detail below) as being a mechanism for AR activation and localisation in the absence of the ligand. Through the use of MAPK pathway inhibitors (p38 MAPK, SB203580; ERK1/2 PD98059; JNK SP600125), total

AR and AR phosphorylation response to IGF-I was blocked. Through a near identical approach, yet addressing the Pi3K/Akt pathway (inhibitor LY294002) similar results were seen by Lee [65] suggesting that both MAPK and PI3K/Akt pathways stimulate AR activity and as these pathways have been shown to be involved in proliferation (MAPK) and differentiation (PI3K/Akt) [68]. Therefore, in conjunction with Testosterone binding to AR to initiate activation, IGF-I also activates AR through the MAPK and Pi3K/Akt pathways suggesting a dual regulation of AR through previously distinct pathways. The activation/synergist behaviour by testosterone on IGF-I may facilitate competition between Testosterone binding directly to AR or increased IGF-I levels activating the AR first, in a ligand-independent manner. Of course, the suggestion of this particular mechanism has only been illustrated within C2C12 skeletal muscle cell lines and thus further evidence in primary muscle cells is warranted to help substantiate these results.

The utilisation of animal models has further allowed research to address the role which T may play in the activation/mediation of IGF-I and its downstream pathways [54, 56]. Yin et al. [56] employed a catabolic mouse model (dexamethasone administration) to investigate the effect of T on reversing muscle atrophy. It was observed that T reversed the effects of atrophy via the activation of the IGF-I downstream targets, Akt, GSk-3β and p70S6K (Table 1.). The activation of downstream target p70S6K has further been associated with androgen-mediated muscle hypertrophy in castrated rats [68]. The role of T supplementation in reversing muscle wasting/loss was further supported by Kovacheva et al. [53], where similar to Yin et al. [56] in using a mouse model, T supplementation reversed muscle loss via activation of Akt signalling pathway. However Wu et al. [54] observed no activation of Akt in rat L6 myoblast cultures through T treatment. This contrast in results highlights a possible factor to be considered. Perhaps the environment of a monolayer culture verses an *in vivo* model, with a subsequent lack of biomimicity maybe causing the discrepancy and requires muscle cells to be placed in current 3-Dimensional (3D) skeletal muscle constructs [70] as highlighted by Sharples and Stewart [55].

The exact mechanisms for T-induced hypertrophy to occur through IGF-I remain controversial due to recent research suggesting that the IGF-I /Growth hormone axis is not necessary to mediate the effects of T on skeletal muscle *in-vitro* [60]. Testosterone was observed by Serra et al. [60] to rescue muscle-specific mass in the absence of both GH and IGF-I, through use of GH-deficient rats that also show suppressed IGF-I levels. A possible explanation for this observation may be due to mTOR, a key regulator of satellite cell growth and proliferation [71]. Previously the use of rapamycin, an inhibitor of mTOR, blocked the overload and IGF-I induced skeletal muscle *in-vivo* and *in-vitro* respectively [57, 72]. The activity of mTOR has been observed to play a key role in mediating the effects of T-induced muscle hypertrophy, independently of IGF-I and Akt after mechanical stimulation [54, 58, 59].

In rat L6 myoblasts, Wu et al. [54] utilised various inhibitors for mTOR, AR, IGF-I and its receptor (IGF-IR) as well as inhibitors for Akt and Erk to address their roles in T-induced hypertrophy. The authors observed that Erk and mTOR play an important role in hypertrophy occurring through T with both being activated under this stimulus. The activation of mTOR and Erk by T administration was observed independently of IGF-I, as the inhibition of IGF-I and IGF-IR still lead to the phosphorylation of mTOR and Erk. The increased activation of mTOR, may further be attributed to T's action on REDD1 (inhibitor of mTOR) which has been observed to have reduced protein levels upon T's administration [73].

Table 1. Various androgen treatments and their interactions with the downstream targets of IGF-I signalling pathway

Signalling Proteins	Published Papers	Androgen Treatment	Activation Level	Target Cells
IGF-IR	Wu et al. [54]	100 nM T	No effect.	Rat L6 myoblasts
MAPK	Kovacheva et al. [53]	0.5cm or 1.0cm T Implant	No effect.	Young vs. Old Mice
	Brown et al. [74]	2cm T Implant	↑	Mouse Model.
ERK 1/2	Wu et al. [54]	100nM T	↑	Rat L6 myoblasts
	Brown et al. [74]	2cm T Implant	No effect.	Mouse Model
Akt	Yin et al. [56]	0.5 mg/100g/day T	↑	Rat Model
	Wu et al. [54]	100 nM T	No effect.	Rat L6 myoblasts
	Kovacheva et al. [53]	0.5 or 1.0cm T implant	↑	Young vs. Old Mice
mTOR	Wu et al. [54]	100 nM T	↑	Rat L6 myoblasts
p70s6k	Yin et al. [56]	0.5 mg/100g/day T	No effect.	Rat model
	Xu et al. [69]	0.3mg/kg or 3.0mg/kg DHT	↑	Rat model (Castrated)
	Wu et al. [54]	100nM T	↑	Rat L6 myoblasts
GSk-3β	Yin et al. [56]	0.5 mg/100g/day T	↑	Rat model
	Gentile et al. [43]	3mg/kg per day DHT	↑	Rat model (Castrated)

In opposition to findings of Wu et al. [54], Brown et al. [74] observed no activation within Erk in T supplementation of a mouse model, suggesting varying results between cell lines and *in-vivo* models. Thus further investigation is warranted with other cell lines and *in-vivo* experimentation to see if T-induced hypertrophy is dependent on Erk and mTOR activity. To note, IGF-IR and Akt were not activated by T, highlighted through no increases in expression and protein content in rat L6 myoblasts. The inactivation of IGF-IR may aid in the evidence for IGF-I not mediating the effects of T, as Wu et al. [54] observed unaltered changes in IGF-I mRNA levels with T administration.

MAPK/JNK/Notch Signalling

As previously mentioned, Mitogen-activated protein kinases (MAPK's) are another family of downstream proteins activated by IGF-I (Figure 4.) and consists of three subfamilies, ERK (1/2), p38 MAPK and JNK [66, 74]. ERK (1/2) is activated in response to a growth stimuli and thus involved in promoting cell growth where as p38 MAPK and JNK are involved in growth inhibition and promoting apoptosis (cell death) through either inflammatory or environmental signals [74].However, p38 MAPK has dual roles and has been implicated as a differentiation regulator with different isoforms having distinct functions. Where p38-α promotes differentiation and inhibis proliferation where as p38-β hasthe opposite actions on activated satellite cells [75]. Testosterone supplementation has been observed to influence all these proteins in inducing muscle fibre hypertrophy and rescuing muscle mass size in an aging model [53, 74]. More specifically, Brown et al. [74] utilised a mouse model of T-induced hypertrophy where it was observed that after 2-4 weeks of T supplementation (Table 2.), p38 MAPK was activated (high levels of phosphorylated p38 MAPK) and JNK inhibited (decreased levels of phosphorylated JNK). Kovacheva et al. [53] further supported these observations using the same mouse model. Notch signalling represents another alternative pathway as the pathway is responsible for the activation, proliferation and the myogenic progression of satellite cells [76, 77]. Thus testosterone supplementation may increase satellite cell number via the activation of this pathway. T has indeed been observed to increase the expression of Delta, the ligand which binds to activate the Notch receptor [74]. Notch signalling is mediated via the activation of p38 MAPK, which has been observed to be induced through a T stimulus in young mice [74]. Using inhibitors for p38 MAPK [74] highlighted a reduction in the activation of Notch signalling in the presence of T. The impact of reduced Notch signalling resulted in decreased expression of Notch 1 and Notch 2 as well as decreased expression of myogenin (muscle specific transcription factor and promoter of expression of creatine kinase and cytoskeletal proteins e.g. titin and desmin. As the increase in all these factors resulted in muscle fibre hypertrophy, it may be suggested that p38 MAPK can activate Notch signalling contributing to hypertrophy via a T stimulus. In comparison, T appeared not to activate p38 MAPK in aged mice. However, through the increased expression of Notch 1, T still reversed age-related effects on skeletal muscle i.e. decreased the levels of myostatin and increased inhibition of JNK contributing to rescuing muscle mass size [53]. Therefore, it may be suggested that the signalling pathways mediating this process may vary with age per se or p38 MAPK is not fundamental in T action which may suggest an alternative mechanism maybe more important.

Wnt/β –Catenin Signalling

Wnt signalling consists of Wingless and Int, a family of secreted glycoproteins [78]. This particular pathway is responsible for the regulation of cell cycle control and cell-cell adhesion [79]. The effects of Wnt are mediated via β-catenin signalling, once Wnt has been activated. This activation leads to the translocation of β-Catenin into the nuclei and the regulation of target genes, through its binding to T-cell factor (TCF) and lymphoid-enhancing factor (LEF) [78, 79]. Furthermore, β-catenin forms a complex with the AR [80] and therefore suggests potential cross talk between β-catenin and AR signalling (Figure 2.). This has indeed been observed under T treatment to activate β-catenin's translocation into the nucleus of mouse cells [80] and of cattle [78]. Subsequently this pathway has been observed to play a role within myogenesis, with T treatment inducing a heightened response [78, 80]. Through the treatment of trenbolone, Zhao et al. [78] observed increases in cellular β-catenin levels and that β-catenin formed a complex with the androgen receptor enhancing myogenesis in muscle-derived stem cells from cattle. Furthermore, adenosine monophosphate-activated protein kinase (AMPK) appeared to stabilise β-catenin levels through the trenbolone stimulus, adding evidence for an alternative mechanism in T promoting myogenesis within skeletal muscle cells.

Gentile et al. [43] utilised a castrated rat model to identify potential downstream effectors and genes involved in the anabolic actions of androgens (DHT and T) after 21 days of treatment. Most notably, AXIN 1 and AXIN 2 were down-regulated by DHT plus serine-9 phosporylation of GSK-3β, resulting in the inhibition of GSK-3β, factors which contribute to β-catenin signalling activation. The Wnt/β-Catenin pathway may further play a role in hypertrophy, through increased gene expression of c-Myc and Cyclin D1, which are involved in cell cycle regulation and the regulation of cell size [81, 82]. The use of Nandrolone decanoate (anabolic steroid) treatment has been observed to induce Cyclin D1 expression as well as the suppression of p21 and myogenin mRNA in rat soleus muscle [83]. Thus an important consideration maybe whether endogenous T is involved more in promoting proliferation of muscle cells or promoting myogenesis as increased cyclin D would promote cycling through S/G2 phases of the cell cycle and without adequate cyclin dependant kinase inhibitor p21 and myogenin expression would reduce the ability of the cells to exit the cell cycle in G1, a prerequisite for myoblast differentiation. Therefore, future research may focus on the role of other characteristics involved downstream of Wnt/β-catenin signalling, as an impact of its activation due to T.

Myostatin/TGF-β Signalling

The molecular mechanism for how T-induces the promotion of muscle growth and hypertrophy is one aspect considered so far. An alternative aspect to consider is the possible role of action testosterone exerts on pathways (Table 2.) involved in growth inhibition, protein degradation and programmed cell death (apoptosis). Transforming growth factor-β (TGF-β) signalling pathway is responsible for the inhibition of myogenic differentiation [84]. Follistatin is a Wnt target gene, expressed following β-catenin nuclear localisation and subsequently plays a role in binding to TGF-β family members. One such family member is myostatin and thus Follistatin inhibits the activity of myostatin (endogenous inhibitor of growth) [85]. Myostatin is responsible for the up-regulation of p21, an inhibitor of cyclin-dependant kinase (CDK) and subsequently cell cycle withdrawl in G1 and thus differentiation with the subsequent inhibition of cell proliferation [53, 86]. In addition, myostatin has been observed to reduce myotube size and differentiation of myoblasts via Akt/mTOR and p70S6K signalling (pathways suggested to be activated by T) [87].

Testosterone supplementation has been observed to down-regulate the expression of myostatin [53, 88]. Through the suggested AR/β-Catenin cross talk leading to the expression of Wnt target genes, follistatin is up-regulated following T administration and thus the regulation of TGF-β signalling [74].

Furthermore, T inhibits JNK [74], which besides MAPK interaction with T, is a possible consequence of the reduction in myostatin expression.

Table 2. The interaction of Androgens with alternative (growth inhibition/cell development) signalling pathways

Protein	Published Paper	Androgen treatment	Activation Level	Target Cells
Myostatin	Mendler et al. [88]	T propionate 100ug/100g body weight for 4 weeks	↓	Male Wister rats (Castrated)
JNK	Brown et al. [74] Kovacheva et al. [53]	2cm T Implant 0.5cm/1.0cm T Implants	↓ ↓	Mouse Model Young vs. Old Mice
Notch 1 and 2	Brown et al. [74]	2cm T Implant	Increased expression after 1 & 8 weeks.	Mouse Model
Delta	Brown et al. [74]	2cm T Implant	Increased expression after 2 and 8 weeks	Mouse Model
β-Catenin	Singh et al. [80] Gentile et al. [43]	100nM T & 10nM DHT 3mg/kg per day DHT.	↑ Plus translocation to the nucleus. Acute increase after 1-7 days.	Mouse C3H 10T1/2 cells Rat Model (Castrated)
Cyclin D1	McClung et al. [83]	6mg/kg body weight, Nandrolone Decanoate	↓ mRNA levels.	Rat soleus muscle
REDD1	Wu et al. [73]	28mg/kg/day and 100-500nM T	↓ Protein and mRNA expession	Dexamethasone - treated rats & rat L6.AR myoblasts
4E-BP-1	Wu et al. [73]	28mg/kg/day T	↓	
FOXO1	Qin et al. [89]	28mg/kg/day T	↓	
MAFbx	Zhao et al. [91]	28mg/kg/day T	↓ mRNA levels.	

The inactivation of JNK may further play a role through stimulating cellular proliferation by reducing the up-regulation of p21 [89]. These potential events influenced by T may offer a potential mechanism of action for T through a reduction in cell apoptosis causing increased cell growth instead. Therefore with age, T's action may be a protective function [90, 91], that is more specific towards sarcopenia and muscle wasting diseases, where metabolites associated with grown inhibition, reduced regenerative capacity and cell apoptosis are highly expressed [92].

TESTOSTERONE AND CALCIUM CONCENTRATION

To underpin how limited our understanding of T is, it is worth noting the additional effects of T on skeletal muscle cells tha have been investigated. In addition to the classical genomic (functional effect on the cells through gene regulation) actions of T, research has attempted to address the non-genomic (rapid) actions too. The alteration in protein synthesis highlights the genomic action, with the process taking hours to days where as the non-genomic action of testosterone is from seconds to minutes within skeletal muscle [93]. A concept of testosterone's rapid action involves the increase in intracellular Ca^{2+} [94, 95]. The increase in Ca2+ has been observed to increase the phosphorylation of ERK (1/2) [96]. Hamdi and Mutungi [96] observed that T had no effect on maximum isometric force in both slow and fast twitch fibres of isolated intact mouse skeletal muscle. However, T's derivate, DHT was observed to increase force in fast twitch fibres, yet decreased in slow twitch fibres. Furthermore DHT activated ERK (1/2) in both fibre types, where as T only activated ERK (1/2) in slow twitch fibres. Therefore, it may be suggested that T's action is involved around genomic pathways, yet its conversion to DHT may influence more non-genomic actions in skeletal muscle. Yet further research is warranted to ascertain more evidence for non-genomic actions of T on skeletal muscle.

EXPERIMENTAL CONSIDERATIONS

Although recent research has begun to address various possible pathways which testosterone may mediate and activate skeletal muscle hypertrophy, the mechanisms and time course of these molecular events triggered by T remain inconclusive and frequently contradictory.. Potential reasons for inconclusive and contrasting results revolve around factors in experimental approaches utilised. The adoption of muscle cells lines vs. primary human culture to address cell behaviour may facilitate different responses to androgen treatment with respect to myoblast proliferation and differentiation capacity [60]. Even the comparison between muscle cells of the same species is difficult with varying androgen-responsiveness in muscle itself [97-99]. Culture systems are commonly monolayer, yet within the body, cell-cell and cell-matrix interactions occur within a 3-D environment. The role of the vascular network in skeletal muscle is another factor which limits current monolayer and 3D culture. Another limit is the lack of various other cell types, such as fibroblasts and motor neurons, which may play a role in skeletal muscle androgen-responsiveness [60, 99]. Most notably, as this chapter has attempted to highlight, is the complexity of a human organism and thus any experimental model would struggle to replicate this fact [60]. The best scenario would be a physiological tool to bridge the gap between conventional 2-D culture systems and *in-vivo* models [100].

FUTURE DIRECTIONS/CONCLUSION

Various pathways have been addressed within the literature for which T may influence directly (Androgen receptor) or indirectly (IGF-I, mTOR MAPK, β-Catenin etc.) or interaction between IGF-I and AR to promote muscle growth and hypertrophy. However, more evidence, using either *in-vitro* or *in-vivo* models, on these various pathways are required to assess the contribution of each pathway in muscle growth/hypertrophy under a T stimulus. Such evidence would allow for a more complete understanding of the action of T. The future applications of T administration, synthetic derivatives and SARMs in the treatment of sarcopenia and muscle wasting diseases can be harnessed based on the identified mechanism [4].

Finally, engineered skeletal muscle represents a potential tool for investigating both physiology and function of muscle [100]. The utilisation of such 3-D models can aid in our understanding of molecular aspects involved in muscle force generation, adaptation, repair and regeneration [70, 100]. Tissue-engineered muscle would further enable us to address the influences of various stimuli on muscle such as the aging process and responses to exercise [101]. Of course, not to discredit current experimental approaches as monolayer *in-vitro* models can be still implemented to answer key molecular regulation, yet through engineering strategies, these models could be more reflective of the *in-vivo* environment [55].

REFERENCES

[1]   Bashin, S., Storer, T.W., Berman, N., Callegari, C., Clevenger, B., Phillips, J., et al. (1996). The effects of supraphysiologic doses of

testosterone on muscle size and strength in normal men. *The New England Journal of Medicine, 335,* 1-7.

[2]   Evans, N.A. (2004). Current concepts in anabolic-androgenic steroids. *The American Journal of Sports Medicine, 32,* 534-542.

[3]   Hartgens, F. and Kuipers, H. (2004). *Effects of androgenic-anabolic steroids in athletes. Sports Medicine, 34,* 513-554.

[4]   Dillon, E.L., Durham, W.J., Urban, R.J. and Sheffield-Moore, M. (2010). Hormone treatment and muscle anabolism during aging: Androgens. *Clinical Nutrition, 29,* 697-700.

[5]   Sinha-Hikim, I., Roth, S.M., Lee, M.I. and Bashin, S. (2003). Testosterone-induced muscle hypertrophy is associated with an increase in satellite cell number in healthy, young men. *American Journal of Physiology Endocrinology and Metabolism,* 285, 197-205.

[6]   Traish, M.A., Miner, M.M., Morgentaler, A., and Zitzmann, M. (2011). Testosterone Deficiency. *The American Journal of Medicine, 124, 578-587.*

[7]   Sattler, F., Bashin, S., Hue, J., Chou, C., Castenada-Sceppa, C., Yarasheski, K., et al. (2011). Testosterone threshold levels and lean tissue mass targets needed to ehance skeletal muscle strength and function: The HORMA trial. *Journal of Gerontology: Medical Sciences, 66A,* 122-129.

[8]   Ting, H.J. and Chang, C. (2008). Actin associated proteins function as androgen receptor coregulators: An implication of androgen receptor's role in skeletal muscle. *Journal of Steroid Biochemistry and Molecular Biology, 111,* 157-163.

[9]   Kim, H. (2007). Regulation of gonadotropin-releasing hormone gene expression. *Seminars in Reproductive Medicine, 25,* 313-325.

[10] Vingren, J.L., Kraemer, W.J., Ratamess, N.A., Anderson, J.M., Volek, J.S. and Maresh, C.M. (2010). Testosterone physiology in resistance training: The up-stream regulatory elements. *Sports Medicine, 40,* 1037-1063.

[11] Miller, W.L. (1988). Molecular biology of steroid hormone synthesis. *Endocrine Reviews, 9,* 295-318.

[12] Payne, A.H. and Hales, D.B. (2004). Overview of steroidogenic enzymes in the pathway from cholesterol to active steroid hormones. *Endocrine Reviews, 25, 947-970.*

[13] Labrie, F. (1991). Intracrinology. *Molecular and Cellular Endocrinology, 78,* 113-118.

[14] Luu-The, V. and Labrie, F. (2010). The intracrine sex steroid biosynthesis pathways. *Progress in Brain Research, 181,* 177-192.

[15] Vandenput, L. and Ohlsson, C. (2010). Sex steroid metabolism in the regulation of bone health in men. *Journal of Steroid Biochemistry and Molecular Biology, 121,* 582-588.

[16] Wierman, M.E. (2007). Sex steroid effects at target tissues: mechanisms of action. *Advances in Physiology Education, 31, 26-33.*

[17] Sato, K., Iemitsu, M., Aizawa, K., and Ajisaka, R. (2008). Testosterone and DHEA activate glucose metabolism-related signaling pathway in skeletal muscle. *Journal of American Physiology Endocrinology and Metabolism, 294, 961-968.*

[18] Aizawa, K., Lemitsu, M., Maeda, S., Otsuki, T., Sato, K., Ushida, T., Mesaki, N., and Akimoto, T. (2010). Acute exercise activates local bioactive androgen metabolism in skeletal muscle. *Steroids, 75, 219-223.*

[19] Bennett, N.C., Gardiner, R.A., Hooper, J.D., Johnson, D.W. and Gobe, G.C. (2010). Molecular cell biology of androgen receptor signalling. *The International Journal of Biochemistry and Cell Biology,* 42, 813-827.

[20] Chen, Y., Zajac, J.D. and Maclean, H.E. (2005). Androgen regulation of satellite cell function. *Journal of Endocrinology, 186,* 21-31.

[21] Saartok, T., Dahlberg, E. and Gustafsson, J.A. (1984). Relative binding affinity of androgenic-anabolic steroids: Comparison of the binding to the androgen receptors in skeletal muscle and in prostate, as well as to sex hormone-binding globulin. *Endocrinology, 114,* 2100-2106.

[22] Borst, S.E., Conover, C.F., Carter, C.S., Gregory, C.M., Marzetti, E., Leeuwenburgh, C., et al. (2007). Anabolic effects of testosterone are preserved during inhibition of 5-α reductase. *Journal of American Physiology Endocrinology and Metabolism, 293,* 507-514.

[23] Gennari, L., Merlotti, D., Martini, G., Gonnelli, S., Franci, B., Campagna, S., et al. (2003). Longitudinal association between sex hormone levels, bone loss, and bone turnover in elderly men. *The Journal of Clinical Endocrinology and Metabolism, 88,* 5327-5333.

[24] Kholsa, S., Melton III, L.J., Robb, R.A., Camp, J.J., Atkinson, E.J., Oberg, A.L., et al. (2005). Relationship of volumetric BMD and structural parameters at different skeletal sites to sex steroid levels in men. *Journal of Bone and Mineral Research, 20,* 730-740.

[25] Fink, H.A., Ewing, S.K., Ensrud, K.E., Barrett-Connor, E., Taylor, B.C., Cauley, J.A., et al. (2006). Association of testosterone and estradiol

deficiency with osteoporosis and rapid bone loss in older men. *The Journal of Clinical Endocrinology and Metabolism, 91*, 3908-3915.

[26] Ward, K.A., Pye, S.R., Adams, J.E., Boonen, S., Vanderschueren, D., Borghs, H., et al. (2011). Influence of age and sex steroids on bone density and geometry in middle-aged and elderly European men. *Osteoporosis International, 22*, 1513-1523.

[27] Callewaert, F., Boonen, S. and Vanderschueren, D. (2010). Sex steroids and the male skeleton: A tale of two hormones. *Trends in Endocrinology and Metabolism, 21*, 89-95.

[28] Ahtiainen, J., Hulmi, J., Kraemer, W., Lehti, M., Nyman, K., Selanne, H., et al. (2011). Heavy resistance exercise training and skeletal muscle androgen receptor expression in younger and older men. *Steroids, 76*, 183-192.

[29] Brodsky, I.G., Balagopal, P. and Nair, K.S. (1996). Effects of testosterone replacement on muscle mass and muscle protein synthesis in hypogonadal men-a clinical research center study. *The Journal of Clinical Endocrinology and Metabolism, 81*, 3469-3475.

[30] Sheffield-Moore, M., Urban, R.J., Wolfe, S.E., Jiang, J., Catlin, D.H., Herndon, D.N., et al. (1999). Short-term oxandrolone administration stimulates net muscle protein synthesis in young men. *The Journal of Clinical Endocrinology and Metabolism, 84*, 2705-2711.

[31] Bashin, S., Woodhouse, L., Casaburi, R., Singh, A.B., Bashin, D., Berman, N., et al. (2001). Testosterone dose-response relationships in healthy young men. *American Journal of Physiology Endocrinology and Metabolism, 281*, 1172-1181.

[32] Sinha-Hikim, I., Artaza, J., Woodhouse, L., Gonzalez-Cadavid, N., Singh, A.B., Lee, M.I., et al. (2002). Testosterone-induced increase in muscle size in healthy young men is associated with muscle fiber hypertrophy. *American Journal of Physiology Endocrinology and Metabolism, 283*, E154-E164.

[33] Kadi, F. and Thornell, L. (2000). Concomitant increases in myonuclear and satellite cell content in female trapezius muscle following strength training. *Histochemistry and Cell Biology, 113*, 99-103.

[34] Eriksson, A., Kadi, F., Malm, C. and Thornell, L. (2005). Skeletal muscle morphology in power-lifters with and without anabolic steroids. *Histochemistry and Cell Biology, 124*, 167-175.

[35] Ferrando, A., Sheffield-Moore, M., Yeckel, C., Gilkison, C., Jiang, J., Achacosa, A., et al. (2002). Testosterone administration to older men improves muscle function: Molecular and physiological mechanisms.

American Journal of Physiology Endocrinology and Metabolism, 282, E601-E607.

[36] Kvorning, T., Andersen, M., Brixen, K., Schjerling, P., Suetta, C. and Madsen, K. (2007). Suppression of testosterone does not blunt mRNA expression of myoD, myogenin, IGF, myostatin or androgen receptor post strength training in humans. *Journal of Physiology, 578,* 579-593.

[37] Inoue, K., Yamasaki, S., Fushiki, T., Okada, Y. and Sugimoto, E. (1994). Androgen receptor antagonist suppresses exercise-induced hypertrophy of skeletal muscle. *European Journal of Applied Physiology, 69,* 88-91.

[38] Masiello, D., Cheng, S., Bubley, G.J., Lu, M.L. and Balk, S.P. (2002). Bicalutamide functions as an androgen receptor antagonist by assembly of a transcriptionally inactive receptor. *The Journal of Biological Chemistry, 277,* 26321-26326.

[39] Maclean, H.E., Chiu, W.S., Notini, A.J., Axell, A.M., Davey, R.A., McManus, J.F., et al. (2008). Impaired skeletal muscle development and function in male, but not female, genomic androgen receptor knockout mice. *The FASEB Journal, 22,* 2676-2689.

[40] Ophoff, J., Proeyen, K.V., Callewaert, F., Gendt, K.D., De Bock, K., Bosch, A.V., et al. (2009). Androgen signaling in myocytes contributes to the maintenance of muscle mass and fiber type regulation but not to muscle strength or fatigue. *Endocrinology, 150,* 3558-3566.

[41] Spiering, B.A., Kraemer, W.J., Vingren, J.L., Ratamess, N.A., Anderson, J.M., Armstrong, L.E., et al. (2009). Elevated endogenous testosterone concentrations potentiate muscle androgen receptor responses to resistance exercise. *Journal of Steroid Biochemistry and Molecular Biology, 114,* 195-199.

[42] Kadi, F. (2008). Cellular and molecular mechanisms responsible for the action of testosterone on human skeletal muscle. A basis for illegal performance enhancement. *British Journal of Pharmacology, 154,* 522-528.

[43] Gentile, M.A., Nantermet, P.V., Vogel, R.L., Phillips, R., Holder, D., Hodor, P., et al. (2010) Androgen-mediated improvement of body composition and muscle function involves a novel early transcription program including IGF1, mechano growth factor, and induction of β-catenin. *Journal of Molecular Endocrinology, 44,* 55-73.

[44] Gobinet, J., Poujol, N. and Sultan, C. (2002). Molecular action of androgens. *Molecular and Cellular Endocrinology, 198,* 15-24.

[45] Wannenes, F., Caprio, M., Gatta, L., Fabbri, A., Bonini, S. and Moretti, C. (2008). Androgen receptor expression during C2C12 skeletal muscle cell line differentiation. *Molecular and Cellular Endocrinology*, 292, 11-19.

[46] Lee, D. (2002). Androgen receptor enhances myogenin expression and accelerates differentiation. *Biochemical and Biophysical Research Communications*, 294, 408-413.

[47] Sinha-Hikim, I., Taylor, W.E., Gonzalez-Cadavid, N.F., Zheng, W. and Bhasin, S. (2004). Androgen receptor in human skeletal muscle and cultured muscle satellite cells: Up-regulation by androgen treatment. *The Journal of Clinical Endocrinology and Metabolism*, 89, 5245-5255.

[48] Kadi, F., Charifi, N., Denis, C., Lexell, J., Andersen, J., Schjerling, P., et al. (2005). The behaviour of satellite cells in response to exercise: What have we learned from human studies? *Pflugers Archive European Journal of Physiology*, 451, 319-327.

[49] Sinanan, A.C.M., Buxton, P.G., and Lewis, M.P. (2006). Muscling in on stem cells. *Biology of the Cell*, 98, 203-214.

[50] Kadi, F., Eriksson, A., Holmner, S., Butler-Browne, G.S. and Thornell, L. (1999). Cellular adaptation of the trapezius muscle in strength-trained athletes. *Histochemistry and Cell Biology*, 111, 189-195.

[51] Vingren, J.L., Kraemer, W.J., Hatfield, D.L., Volek, J.S., Ratamess, N.A., Anderson, J.M., et al. (2009). Effect of resistance exercise on muscle steroid receptor protein content in strength-trained men and women. *Steroids*, 74, 1033-1039.

[52] Ratamess, N.A., Kraemer, W.J., Volek, J.S., Maresh, C.M., Vanheest, J.L., Sharman, M.J., et al. (2005). Androgen receptor content following heavy resistance exercise in men. *Journal of Steroid Biochemistry and Molecular Biology*, 93, 35-42.

[53] Kovacheva, E.L., Hikim, A.M.S., Shen, R., Shinha, I. and Sinha-Hikim, I. (2010). Testosterone supplementation reverses sarcopenia in aging through regulation of myostatin, c-jun NH_2 Terminal kinase, notch, and akt signaling pathways. Endocrinology, 151, 628-638.

[54] Wu, Y., Bauman, W.A., Blitzer, R.D. and Cardozo, C. (2010). Testosterone-induced hypertrophy of L6 myoblasts is dependent upon erk and mTOR. *Biochemical and Biophysical Research Communications*, 400, 679-683.

[55] Sharples, A.P. and Stewart, C.E. (2011). Myoblast models of skeletal muscle hypertrophy and atrophy. *Current Opinion in Clinical Nutrition and Metabolic Care*, 14, 230-236.

[56] Yin, H., Chai, J., Yu, Y., Shen, C., Wu, Y., Yao, Y., et al. (2009). Regulation of signalling pathways downstream of IGF-I/Insulin by androgen in skeletal muscle of glucocorticoid-treated rats. *The Journal of Trauma*, *66*, 1083-1090.

[57] Rommel, C., Bodine, S., Clarke, B., Rossman, R., Nunez, L., Stitt, T., et al. (2001). Mediation of IGF-I induced skeletal myotube hypertrophy by PI(3)K/Akt/mTOR and PI(3)/Akt/GSK3 pathways. *Nature Cell Biology*, *3*, 1009-1013.

[58] Miyazaki, M., McCarthy, J.J., Fedele, M.J., and Esser, K.A. (2011). Early activation of mTORC1 signalling in response to mechanical overload is independent of phosphoinositide 3-kinase/Akt signalling. *Journal of Physiology*, *589*, *1831-1846.*

[59] Spangenburg, E.E., Le Roith, D., Ward, C.W., and Bodine, S.C. (2008). A functional insulin-like growth factor receptor is not necessary for load-induced skeletal muscle hypertrophy. *Journal of Physiology*, *586*, *283-291.*

[60] Serra, C., Bashin, S., Tangherlini, F., Barton, E., Ganno, M., Zhang, A., et al. (2011). The role of GH and IGF-I in mediating anabolic effects of testosterone on androgen-responsive muscle. *Endocrinology*, *152*, 193-206.

[61] Sculthorpe, N., Solomon, A.M., Sinanan, A.C.M., Bouloux, P.M.G., Grace, F., and Lewis, M.P. (2011). Androgens affect myogenesis *in vitro* in association with increased local IGF-I. Medicine and Science in Sports and Exercise[Epub ahead of print] Pubmed PMID: 21946153.

[62] Ates, K., Yang, S.Y., Orrell, R.W., Sinanan, A.C.M., Simons, P., Solomon, A., Beech, S., Goldspink, G., and Lewis, M.P. (2007). The IGF-I splice variant MGF increases progenitor cells in ALS, Dystrophic, and normal muscle. *FEBS letters*, *581*, *2727-2732.*

[63] Hill, M. and Goldspink, G. (2003). Expression and spicing of the insulin-like growth factor gene in rodent muscle is associated with muscle satellite (stem) cell activation following local tissue damage. *The Journal of Physiology*, *549*, 409-418.

[64] Hammed, M., Orrell, R.W., Cobbold, M., Goldspink, G., and Harridge, S.D.R. (2003). Expression of IGF-I splice variants in young and old human skeletal muscle after high resistance exercise. *Journal of Physiology*, *547*, *247-254.*

[65] Lee, W. (2009). Insulin-like growth factor-I induced androgen receptor activation is mediated by the PI3/Akt pathway in C2C12 skeletal muscle cells. *Molecules and Cells*, *28*, 495-499.

[66] Kim, H. and Lee, W. (2009). Insulin-like growth factor-I induces androgen receptor activation in differentiating C2C12 skeletal muscle cells. *Molecules and Cells*, *28*, 189-194.

[67] Kim, H. and Lee, W. (2009). Ligand-independant activation of the androgen receptor by insulin-like growth factor-I and the role of MAPK pathway in skeletal muscle cells. *Molecules and Cells*, *28*, 589-593.

[68] Coolican, S.A., Samuel, D.S., Ewton, D.Z., McWade, F.J. and Florini, J.R. (1997). The mitogenic and myogenic actions of insulin-like growth factors utilize distinct signalling pathways. *The Journal of Biological Chemistry*, *272*, 6653-6662.

[69] Xu, T., Shen, Y., Pink, H., Triantafillou, J., Stimpson, S.A., Turnbull, P., et al. (2004). Phosphorylation of p70S6 kinase is impacted in androgen-induced levator ani muscle anabolism in castrated rats. *Journal of Steroid Biochemistry and Molecular Biology*, *92*, 447-454.

[70] Mudera, V., Smith, A.S.T., Brady, M.A. and Lewis, M.P. (2010). The effect of cell density on the maturation and contractile ability of muscle derived cells in a 3-D tissue-engineered skeletal muscle model and determination of the cellular and mechanical stimuli required for the synthesis of a postural phenotype. *Journal of Cellular Physiology*, *225*, 646-653.

[71] Sarbassov, D.D., Ali, S.M. and Sabatini, D.M. (2005). Growing roles for the mTOR pathway. *Current Opinion in Cell Biology*, *17*, 596-603.

[72] Bodine, S.C., Stitt, T.N., Gonzalez, M., Kline, W.O., Stover, G.L., Bauerlin, R., et al. (2001). Akt/mTOR pathway is a crucial regulator of skeletal muscle hypertrophy and can prevent muscle atrophy in vivo. *Nature Cell Biology*, *3*, 1014-1019.

[73] Wu, Y., Zhao, W., Zhao, J., Zhang, Y., Qin, W., Pan, J., Bauman, W.A., Blitzer, R.D., and Cardozo, C. (2010). REDD1 is a major target of testosterone action in preventing dexamethansone-induced muscle loss. *Endocrinology*, *151*, 1050-1059.

[74] Brown, D., Hikim, A.M.S., Kovacheva, E.L. and Sinha-Hikim, I. (2009). Mouse model of testosterone-induced muscle fiber hypertrophy: Involvement of p38 mitogen-activated protein kinase-mediated notch signaling. *Journal of Endocrinology*, *201*, 129-139.

[75] Lassar, A.B. (2009). The p38 MAPK family, a pushmi-pullyu of skeletal muscle differentiation. *The Journal of Cell Biology*, *187*, 941-943.

[76] Conboy, I.M., Conboy, M.J., Smythe, G.M. and Rando, T.A. (2003). Notch-mediated restoration of regenerative potential to aged muscle. *Science*, *302*, 1575-1577.

[77] Sinha-Hikim, I., Cornford, M., Gaytan, H., Lee, M.L. and Bhasin, S. (2006). Effects of testosterone supplementation on skeletal muscle fiber hypertrophy and satellite cells in community-dwelling older men. *The Journal of Clinical Endocrinology and Metabolism*, *91*, 3024-3033.

[78] Zhao, J.X., Hu, J., Zhu, M.J. and Du, M. (2011). Trenbolone enhances myogenic differentiation by enhancing β-catenin signalling in muscle-derived stem cells of cattle. *Domestic Animal Endocrinology*, *40*, 222-229.

[79] Mulholland, D.J., Dedhar, S., Coetzee, G.A. and Nelson, C.C. (2005). Interaction of the nuclear receptors with the wnt/beta-catenin/tcf signaling axis: Wnt you like to know? *Endocrine Reviews*, *26*, 898-915.

[80] Singh, R., Bashin, S., Braga, M., Artaza, J.N., Pervin, S., Taylor, W.E., et al. (2009). Regulation of myogenic differentiation by androgens: Cross talk between androgen receptor/beta-catenin and follistatin/transforming growth factor-beta signaling pathways. *Endocrinology*, *150*, 1259-1268.

[81] Armstrong, D.D. and Esser, K.A. (2005). Wnt/β-catenin signaling activates growth-control genes during overload-induced skeletal muscle hypertrophy. *American Journal of Physiology Cell Physiology*, *289*, 853-859.

[82] Montagne, J. (2000). Genetic and molecular mechanisms of cell size control. *Molecular Cell Biology Research Communications*, *4*, 195-202.

[83] McClung, J.M., Mehl, K.A., Thompson, R.W., Lowe, L.L. and Carson, J.A. (2005). Nandrolone decanoate modulates cell cycle regulation in functionally overloaded rat soleus muscle. *American Journal of Physiology. Regulatory, Integrative and Comparative Physiology*, *288*, R1543-1552.

[84] Beggs, M.L., Nagarajan, R., Taylor-Jones, J.M., Nolen, G., Macnicol, M. and Peterson, C.A. (2004). Alterations in the TGFβ signaling pathway in myogenic progenitors with age. *Aging Cell*, *3*, 353-361.

[85] Amthor, H., Nicholas, G., McKinnell, I., Kemp, C.F., Sharma, M., Kambadur, R., et al. (2004). Follistatin complexes myostatin and antagonizes myostatin-mediated inhibition of myogenesis. *Developmental Biology*, *270*, 19-30.

[86] McCroskery, S., Thomas, M., Maxwell, L., Sharma, M. and Kambadur, R. (2003). Myostatin negatively regulates satellite cell activation and self-renewal. *The Journal of Cell Biology*, *162*, 1135-1147.

[87] Trendelenburg, A.U., Meyer, A., Rohner, D., Boyle, J., Hatakeyama, S. and Glass, D.J. (2009). Myostatin reduces Akt/TORC1/p70S6K

signalling, inhibiting myoblast differentiation and myotube size. *American Journal of Physiology Cell Physiology, 296,* C1258-C1270.

[88] Mendler, L., Baka, Z., Kovacs-Simon, A. and Dux, L. (2007). Androgens negatively regulate myostatin expression in an androgen-dependant skeletal muscle. *Biochemical and Biophysical Research Communications, 361,* 237-242.

[89] Huang, Z., Chen, D., Zhang, K., Yu, B., Chen, X. and Meng, J. (2007). Regulation of myostatin signalling by c-jun N-terminal kinase in C2C12 cells. *Cellular Signalling, 19,* 2286-2295.

[90] Qin, W., Pan, J., Wu, Y., Bauman, W.A., and Cardozo, C. (2010). Protection against dexamethasone-induced muscle atrophy is related to modulation by testosterone of FOXO1 and PGC1-α. *Biochemical and Biophysical Research Communications, 403,* 473-478.

[91] Zhao, W., Pan, J., Zhao, Z., Wu, Y., Bauman, W.A., and Cardozo, C.P. (2008). Testosterone protects against dexamethasone-induced muscle atrophy, protein degradation and MAFbx upregulation. *Journal of Steroid Biochemistry and Molecular Biology, 110, 125-129.*

[92] Degens, H. (2010). The role of systemic inlfammation in age-related muscle weakness and wasting. *Scandinavian Journal of Medicine and Science in Sports, 20,* 28-38.

[93] Rahman, F. and Christian, H.C. (2007). Non-classical actions of testosterone: An update. *Trends in Endocrinology and Metabolism, 18,* 371-378.

[94] Estrada, M., Espinosa, A., Gibson, C.J., Uhlen, P. and Jaimovich, E. (2005). Capacitative entry in testosterone-induced intracellular calcium oscillations in myotubes. *Journal of Endocrinology, 184,* 371-379.

[95] Estrada, M., Espinosa, A., Muller, M. and Jaimovich, E. (2003). Testosterone stimulates intracellular calcium release and mitogen-activated protein kinases via a G protein-coupled receptor in skeletal muscle cells. *Endocrinology, 144,* 3586-3597.

[96] Hamdi, M.M. and Mutungi, G. (2010). Dihydrotestosterone activates MAPK pathway and modulates maximum isometric force through the EGF receptor in isolated intact mouse skeletal muscle fibres. *Journal of Physiology, 588,* 511-525.

[97] Kadi, F., Bonnerud, P., Eriksson, A. and Thornell, L. (2000). The expression of androgen receptors in human neck and limb muscles: Effects of training and self-administration of androgenic-anabolic steroids. *Histochemistry and Cell Biology, 113,* 25-29.

[98] Johansen, J.A., Breedlove, S.M., and Jordan, C.L. (2007). Androgen receptor expression in the levator anti muscle of male mice. *Journal of Neuroendocrinology*, *19*, 823-826.

[99] Mosler, S., Pankratz, C., Seyfried, A., Piechotta, M., and Diel, P. (2011). The anabolic steroid methandienone targets the hypothalamic-pituitary-testicular axis and myostatin signaling in a rat training model. Archives of Toxicology, DOI: 10.1007/s00204-011-0740-z.

[100] Khodabukus, A., Paxton, J.Z., Donnelly, K. and Baar, K. (2007). Engineered muscle: A tool for studying muscle physiology and function. *Exercise and Sport Science Reviews*, *35*, 186-191.

[101] Passey, S., Martin, N., Player, D. and Lewis, M.P. (2011). Stretching skeletal muscle in vitro: Does it replicate in vivo physiology? *Biotechnology Letters*, 33, 1513-1521.

In: Perspectives on Anabolic Androgenic ….   ISBN: 978-1-62081-243-3
Editors: F. Grace and J. S. Baker   © 2012 Nova Science Publishers, Inc.

Chapter 3

ANABOLIC ANDROGENIC STEROID (AAS) USE – PERSPECTIVES OF A GENERAL PRACTITIONER AND SPORTS PHYSICIAN

Gareth L. Jones

ABSTRACT

This chapter reflects the thought and concerns of a general practitioner and sports physician in relation to the use of anabolic androgenic steroids (AAS). Colleagues in general practice associate their use with the sport of weightlifting, wrestling and bodybuilding in the main [1]. This chapter will summarise the currently available information on AAS use by the sports person and centres on who is using them, reasons for use, supplementation regimens and associated side effects which commonly present at sports clinic and general practice.

As a sports physician, one reads with interest their use in other sports including cycling and occasionally rugby and association football. There is a perception that people who attend bodybuilding gymnasiums have the ambition to maintain positive health and an attractive body shape. A proportion of these individuals' body image perception is distorted somewhat when they present to the general practitioner surgery. The concept of body dysmorphia has become officially recognised. Where women often desire a slim figure, men seem to aspire to larger, toned bodies. Dissatisfaction with their own bodies seems to have increased in recent years [2]. The dissatisfaction with specific regard to muscularity has been described as 'muscle dysmorphia' by some authors [3] although there is some dispute as to whether this is a separate entity to 'body dysmorphia' Their dissatisfaction leads some males to become preoccupied with exercise, particularly weightlifting. This group of males is widely thought to be at risk of both using and misusing anabolic steroids.

There have been many reports on the use of anabolic steroids in high school athletes. Buckley [4]; his colleagues reported a 50.3% questionnaire response, wherein 6.69% of respondents reported current or previous use of steroids, with some declaring they first used steroids at the age of 15 or younger [5]. Interestingly Windsor sent questionnaires to two groups of high school students with a response rate of 92.4% in the affluent student group and 86% in the less affluent group. The affluent group had a 10.2% usage compared to 2.8% usage among the less affluent, the vast majority being male students.

A study by Williamson [6] was the first to report on the use of anabolic steroids among British college students. There was a 92% response rate to the questionnaire with 2.8% reporting current or previous use. Of these 56% reported the use of steroids at the age of 15 yrs or less and 78% at the age of 17 yrs of less. It was interesting that half of the users were rugby players. Improving appearance and physique was the main reason for taking in 39%, improving performance in 28%. Twenty eight percent of the anabolic steroids were obtained on the 'black market', 22% by mail order, 17% from a health professional and 33% unspecified.

The British Crime Survey in 2010, published by the Home Office, estimated that there are 50 000 people in the UK using anabolic steroids to train harder and quickly build muscle. The Advisory Council on the Misuse of Drugs (ACMD) [7] declared that there is an increased use of anabolic steroids by teenagers and med in their twenties to build muscle quickly. The Chairman, Prof Iverson stated that 'the number (using anabolic steroids) for sporting reasons is now a minority' and 'the real growth has come in young users who want to improve their body image'.

Practitioners in this area of medicine believe the majority of competitive athletes have implicitly agreed to a social contract that states:

'We are going to have a fair competition'
'There are things that we can and cannot do'

'Even if anabolic steroids were safe, they may not be available to everybody – using it would still be cheating'

Williamson[6] enquired about what factors would influence them to stop. Sixty two percent would stop if there was an increased risk of a myocardial infarction under the age of 40 yrs, 56% would stop if there was an increased risk of cancer, 55% would stop if there was risk of sterility and 31% would stop if their competitors would stop. This supports the need for education regarding the health risks and the realisation that issues regarding health are more important than 'fair play' – at least among college students in 1993. It is worth posing if this still holds in modern times and would it hold true with the financial reward and notoriety that success brings for the elite athlete?

But, what about the use of anabolic steroids outside the competitive environment?. Is there a public health problem?. Harmer [8] published an article in the BJSM and wondered if the use of anabolic steroids was more of a problem within the general population than in organised sport. He suggested that the public health model was the way to tackle the problem rather than focus on what he felt was more of a sport specific concern such as 'fair play'. In the sport specific model, the 'in competition' and 'out of competition' testing, the threat of suspension or even expulsion if any testing was refused or found to be positive was a 'fear based' approach. This may impact the elite athlete but will significantly less effect the lower level athlete.

Anabolic steroids have been and continue to be used for medical reasons, testosterone replacement therapy in deficiency states and control of metastatic breast cancer. The question arises for what are the perceived benefits to the competitive athlete? In 1993 Korkia and Stimson [9] published an exploratory investigation of 110 users. In order of relative importance, the perceived benefits were:

- 'Increased mass and size'
- 'Increased strength'
- 'Faster recovery from training'
- 'Improved sports performance'
- 'Increased self confidence'
- 'Increased recovery form injury'
- 'Increased aggressiveness'
- 'Decreased body fat'
- 'Other'

Discussion on the evidence behind these perceived benefits is discussed elsewhere, but what are the adverse effects of anabolic steroids? This is an area that has been well documented and been a subject of extensive research. These include adverse effects on the cardiovascular, cerebrovascular, endocrine, hepatocellular, metabolic, dermatological and psychological systems. The precise prevalence of these adverse effects is difficult ascertain because of underreporting.

Exercise results in left ventricular changes commonly resulting in the 'athlete heart'. Amongst the changes seen in power athletes especially is left ventricular hypertrophy. There is some evidence to suggest that use of anabolic steroids in this group of individuals will result in even greater left ventricular hypertrophy [10]. The resulting left ventricular hypertrophy was noted to persist despite the effects of detraining. It is widely accepted that left ventricular hypertrophy is an independent risk factor for cardiac mortality and morbidity.

Asymptomatic left ventricular systolic and diastolic function is also reported after several years of use [11]. In my personal practice, which includes the cardiac screening of international rugby players, echocardiography often displays left ventricular hypertrophy with normal filling patterns (E/A ratio). Echocardiograms performed on anabolic steroid users, restrictive filling patterns are often seen. Systolic heart failure is a common presentation in the older population in general practice and the treatment is well established. Although diastolic heart failure is now well recognised, the optimal treatment has yet to be formulated. Physicians with increasing access to echocardiography, will see an increase in the presentation of diastolic heart failure among long-term users in the future?

The use of anabolic steroids is also associated with an elevation in blood pressure and a reduction in HDL both significant risk factors for flow limiting coronary disease. Reproductive endocrine effects include a loss of libido, although this can increase with small doses. Azoospermia, testicular atrophy and impotence are well-recognised adverse effect. In my experience, gynaecomastia is the most common presentation and in some instance requiring surgery. Virilism can result in females, which in some cases is irreversible. Menstrual irregularity and reversible infertility can result from suppression of the hypothalamic-pituitary-gonadal axis [12] Other effects include glucose intolerance, increased insulin resistance. Increase in benign prostatic hyperplasia resulting in bladder outflow symptoms

Homocysteine is a product form methionine breakdownand is reported to have a detrimental effect on endothelial function by impairing the production of nitric oxide. This results in oxidative stress and the development of atherogenic plaques [13]. A study by Graham [14] in 2006 in ten androgenic steroid users in supraphysiological doses over a period of 20 year did have significantly elevated homocysteine levels. Of the long term users, three had died and they had the higher homocysteine levels of the group. Postmortem examination confirmed a cardiovascular death in each case.

It is accepted that the concentration lipoprotein a (Lp(a)) is an independent risk factor for vascular disease [15]. It appears to be genetically determined so that if elevated, it cannot be lowered by diet or lipid lowering drugs. Anabolic steroids were thought to have a protective effect by lowering Lp(a). A study by Hartgens et al [16] published in 2004 however showed that although a lowering of Lp(a) was found following a polydrug regime of androgenic-anabolic steroids for an eight and fourteen week period. There was also a decrease in t HDL, HDL-2, HDL-3, Apo A1 and Apo-B resulting in an increased atherogenic risk. Prolonged used resulted in a prolonged increase in risk.

Numerous hepatic effects have been documented including cholestasis, peliosis hepatis, benign hepatic tumours associated with high risk of bleeding and malignant change. Peliosis hepatis is the formation of intrahepatic haemorrhagic cysts, which can result in fibrosis. The main concern is that of cyst rupture resulting in a life threatening haemorrhage. Cholestasis will present with an itch and jaundice due to the reduced excretion of bile. Prolonged periods of cholestasis have been reported when anabolic steroids are used in combination with dietary supplements [17]. Such presentations can result in prolonged hospital stays and invasive investigations primarily to exclude other diagnoses. Hepatoma and hepatocellular carcinomas have also been reported but extremely rare [18]. Gorayski et al [19] describes such a case arising in a pre-existing hepatic adenoma. It is uncertain as to whether this transformation from a benign to a malignant lesion was the result of a more recent use of anabolic steroids. This case clearly demonstrated the potential carcinogenic effects of anabolic steroids.

These effects tend to occur following the use of oral anabolic steroids in the main. Other important conditions include hepatitis from needle sharing activities. Hepatic problems are almost exclusively caused by the 17 alpha-alkylated anabolic steroids

The dramatic adverse effects described previously are uncommon, and peliosis hepatis and benign hepatomas can present with perfectly normal liver function tests. Hepatic disorders often present with elevated alanine aminotransferase (ALT), lactate dedydrogenease (LDH) and gamma glutamyl transpeptidase (GGT). It is the ALT that is most often reported in district general hospital together with total bilirubin and alkaline phosphatase. Elevated levels are not always present however physicians would generally be more concerned in those users with elevated liver enzymes.

Adverse renal effects are not often reported but do occur. The use of one performance enhancing drug is often accompanied by the concomitant use of another. The dramatic effects of the use of anabolic steroids together with vetinary sources of vitamin A, D and E was published by Daher [20] and his colleges in 2009. They described two males aged 21 and 31 who presented with abdominal pain and vomiting, biochemical tests showed elevated creatinine and calcium levels. Renal biopsies showed interstitial nephritis and acute tubular necrosis. The authors seem to agree that vitamin D intoxication and anabolic steroid induced interstitial nephritis was responsible for the acute renal dysfunction in both cases although the exact pathophysiology was still to be fully understood.

Dermatological effects could include striae, often in the anterior axillary fold. This may merely relate to the elasticity of the skin not keeping pace with the rapid and recent increase in body shape or bulk. There are few studies that have looked at the possible direct effect on skin elasticity. These striae when associated with other signs, may well be the first indication of anabolic steroid use.

Acne vulgaris is probably the most well recognised side effect of anabolic steroids. This occurs in both male and female users. This is the result of sebaceous cyst hypertrophy. It also associated with an increase in the population of Propionibacteria acnes (P acnes). A study in Finland [21] reported the effects of self administered high dose testosterone and anabolic steroids during a twelve week training period the skin surface lipidsand the P acnes population had significantly increased after eight weeks. This was later confirmed by Scott [22] and his colleagues in 1992 where they also observed an increase in sebaceous cysts, hirsutismandrogenic hair loss pattern, striae, seborrhoeic dermatitis and secondary infections including furunculosis.

The risk of skin and deep abscess is also well recognised among injecting anabolic steroid users. These infections are often attributed to staphylococcus, streptococcus, pseudomonas and mycobacterioun smegmatis. These infections are often the results of needle sharing and therefore could be avoided. Rich et al [23] reported that 60% of needle exchanging programmes reported some anabolic steroid injectors as being part of the programme (512 of 3600 monthly participants). The risks of HIV, hepatitis C and C are also increased in this group. This clearly demonstrated the need to educate those anabolic steroid users who continue to inject.

The recreation use of anabolic steroids is to increase muscle bulk. Some muscle groups are encapsulated within fibrous 'compartments' An increase in pressure within these compartments can have major neuro-vascular effects. Classical compartments are found within the upper and lower limbs. When the pressure within these compartments results in symptoms, decompression is required and in some circumstances this has to be performed as an emergency if the viability of the muscle is to be saved. Anabolic steroids by increasing muscle bulk and their adverse effects on lipid metabolism and resulting atheroma could increase the risk of compartment syndrome.

Acute compartment syndrome is often the result of trauma. Bahia et al [24] reported the case of a body-builder involved in a motorcycle accident who presented with compartment pressure in the upper limbs including areas not normally affected by trauma and wondered whether the use of anabolic steroids contributed to an increased risk of compartment syndrome. This publication should prompt sports physicians to enquire as to the use of anabolic steroids when presented with a case of compartment syndrome.

Anabolic steroids have previously been shown to result in the disorganisation of the tendon fibrillar structure [25] Cases of spontaneous rupture of the extensor policis longus tendon [26], anterior cruciate tendon [27] and quadriceps tendon [28] have been described. Such injuries highlight the imbalance between muscle power and tendon strength. Other factors to consider with regard to musculoskeletal injury are the tendency by anabolic steroid users to train harder for longer, the normal signals such as pain and fatigue being absent or ignored.

Evidence of increased aggression following the use of AAS has been well recognised in power activities but evidence largely anecdotal. As mentioned previously the use of AAS is well recognised in non-competitive individuals. Is there a personality type that is more likely to use AAS? What are the psychological effects on these individuals?

This first question is difficult to answer, as it is very difficult to assess the users personality trait prior to using. Attempts however have been made form historical recall of subjects and comparing data from a group of non-using bodybuilders drawn form the same socioeconomic population matched for age. Copper et al [29]in a study on a group of bodybuilders were able to show that the personality traits of AAS users before the onset of AAS use, assessed retrospectively, were not different from the personality traits of control subjects. They were able to demonstrate a link between significant disturbance in personality profiles and the use of AAS.

Despite this knowledge, some recreational users continue to state:

It hurts only me, so why does society care?'

and because success in sport is associated with fame and financial rewards led to a Canadian sprinter to say:

'The glory is too sweet, the dollars too much'

Some even argue that despite the risks of using anabolic steroids, indeed all perceived performance enhancing drugs, governing bodies and indeed sports physicians continue to tolerate sports that clearly inflict injury such as collision sports. It is difficult to keep all our young people well informed regarding the risks and the benefits of healthy living especially against the well recognised an accepted practice of binge drinking for instance. Such behaviour continues for only a short period and perceived, incorrectly, not to have long lasting effects. Similarly the young anabolic steroid user have also been quoted as using the same argument

'I only take anabolic steroids for a part of my life so what harm can it do'

So how does anabolic user present to the primary care or sports physician and how should we respond?

Anabolic steroid users rarely, if ever, openly admit using at the initial consultation. In the majority of cases in primary care, they present with one or more of the side effects discussed earlier in this chapter. In my experience they are invariably male, acne and gynaecomastia being the most common presentations. On examination, after presentation with a simple chest infection perhaps, striae might be detected. These and other clinical signs might prompt the physician to enquire about the possible current or recent use of anabolic steroids. Denial is often the initial response but after explaining the reason for such an enquiry, a silent acceptance to at least listen to the physicians concerns is the response of many. There are of course those who feel very upset by such direct questioning, such a reaction should in itself raise suspicions.

Today most general practitioners are aware of a 'prohibited list' in sport and the majority, if not all, will be aware that the use of anabolic steroids to enhance performance is on this 'prohibited list'. It is also my experience that most general practitioners will also be aware that competitive athletes are tested in and out of competition. This was not always so, a study published in 1997 [30] found that 12% of general practitioners thought that they were allowed to prescribe anabolic steroids for 'non-medical reasons', 17% did not know. Interestingly 18% had been asked to prescribe anabolic steroids for performance enhancement or body image purposes.

Medical practitioners are often asked to declare 'on line' and complete Therapeutic Exemption forms (TUE) to enable athletes to train and compete whilst taking a substance on the prohibited list. Whilst all sports physicians are aware of this, it is my experience that the general practitioner is not. Athletes should be reminded that it is their responsibility to informin the prescribing physician that they are subject to dope testing. Those physicians uncertain of the prohibited list can check the website www.globaldro.com. If the athlete declares that he is subject to dope testing and asks the prescribing physician to check but fails to do so, or an error was made, then the physician might be deemed to have violated the doping regulation and might be subject to a penalty.

The role of the physician, when presented with a clinical problem related to anabolic steroid use, is to provide the appropriate treatment for the presenting condition. The treatment should include counselling regarding the use of anabolic steroid if this is suspected. The physician should not use 'scare tactics' which could result in loss of the user's confidence and result in the widening of credibility gap between health care professional [31]. The user should clearly be encouraged to stop but the physician is duty bound to provide support and on-going guidance even if the user refuses. The examination should include checking the blood pressure, cardiac examination to look for evidence of left ventricular hypertrophy, testicular examination in males and abdominal examination for hepatomegaly. Evidence of virilisation in women with symptoms such as a deepening voice, hirsutism and male pattern baldness. Routine investigation would include a full blood count, liver function test and lipid profile. Hepatitis and HIV screening would also be advisable for those injecting. It is my usual practice to perform and ECG again looking for evidence of left ventricular hypertrophy on voltage criteria. Clinical assessment for left ventricular hypertrophy is known to have a low degree of sensitivity, as does an ECG but will pick up gross hypertrophy and does send out the correct signals to the user that cardiac problems can and do occur.

In my own practice, the recreational users do take heed of the advice regarding adverse effects and does eventually stop using anabolic steroids. Some have continued however.

In the past Olympic athletes have indeed openly confessed to taking anabolic steroids, Angella Issajenko announced on the 'On the Line' programme on BBC2 in 1989

> 'I came to the conclusion that people I'd compete with in Moscow were also on anabolics, so, I decided that was the way to go. People are not convinced with side effects, or so-called side effects, with anabolic use. They don't believe it. First and foremost what comes to mind is this is going to help ne be the best in the world'

Thankfully this is not the view of the vast majority of today's competitive athlete.

Details of all consultations, as always, should be accurately recorded to include details of all investigations carried out. What if the physician involved is not the user's usual general practitioner? If a competitive athlete consulted a sport's physician and not his registered general practitioner, are there any other issues to be considered?. The sports physician, attached or even employed by a governing body, has responsibilities not only to the athlete but also to the management. In this instance confidentiality becomes a very major and important issue.

The IOC Carter Against Doping in Sports 1989 section 3.3 states that:

> 'Officially appointed national team doctors have the responsibility to advise the team management of possible infringements of the doping regulations of which they are aware'

This raises the conflict between the responsibilities towards and confidentiality of, the athlete and the sports physician's responsibilities towards the governing body and management.

The General Medical Council (GMC) [32] clearly states:

– Make the care of your patient your first concern
– Protect and promote the health of patients and the public
– Respect patient's right to confidentiality

The British Olympic Association in 2000 [33], with specific regard the use of prohibited substances stated that

'Support staff must appreciate that it would be classified as a breech of confidentiality if a member of the medical and scientific support staff revealed that an athletes was taking a prohibited substance, unless the athlete or individual had specifically given consent'

However the World Anti-Doping Code in 2009 stated that if any healthcare professional, according to Article 2.8, is involved in

'..aiding, abetting, covering up or any other type of complicity involving and anti-doping rule violation..'

Then a doping offence is deemed to have occurred. This could then result in the sports physician or other healthcare professional involved being punished.

The GMC have outlined situations where confidentiality could be broken [34]

- In a medical emergency
- Withholding information would put others 'at risk of death or serious harm'
- Those receiving disclosure are bound by confidentiality

These conflicting and important issues are well discussed by McNamee and Phillips [35]. It is clear that the consulting physician should obtain the athlete's written permission prior to forwarding any clinical information to the athlete's general practitioner or any other appropriate healthcare practitioner. If the individual, most likely the recreational user, decides to continue to use anabolic steroids the consulting physician continues to have a duty of care for on-going advise and further monitoring. Sperryn [36] in a paper to the British Association of Sports Medicine Symposium back in 1979 stated that:

'..(the doctor could be) hostile to the management if takes sides with the sportsman'
'..(the doctor could be a) hostile member of the 'Establishment' by the sportsman'

This reminds all sports physicians of the issues involved when dealing with the medical needs of the athlete and the sports governing body he is contracted.

> 'When you are winning a war almost everything that happens can be claimed to be right and wise'
> Winston Churchill

With regard to the use of anabolic steroids for performance enhancing or recreational use, should 'everything' that the individual does, including the use of AAS, considered to be 'right and wise'?

'Dop' was a local liquor of opium used by the African Kaffirs as a stimulant and used for racehorses. The practice of doping has been used by athletes for gaining an advantage over their competitors dating back to the third century when psychotropic mushrooms were used by the Greeks for fighting. In 1865 Dutch canal swimmers were known to use drugs. Syringes and ampoules were found in the locker rooms during the 1952 Oslo Olympic Games. In 1955 French cyclist were tested and five were found to be positive for an undeclared drug.

With evidence of the increased use of drugs the International Olympic Committee (IOC) in 1962 declared a resolution against the use of drugs in sport going on to establish the International Olympic Committee Medical Commission in 1967. The following year 'in competition' testing began.

The Sports Council in 1965 developed a working party looking at the issue of drugs in sport within the UK but King's College London Drug testing centre was not established until 1978. The Sports Council, in 1986, encouraged each sports governing body to start drug testing and agreed to fund such testing.

'Out of competition' testing in the UK did not start until 1981 but only by some governing bodies. The Commonwealth Games Federation also began testing in 1970 but anabolic steroids were not included in the list of prohibited substances. Anabolic steroids is thought to have been used in Olympic competition back in 1960 but it was not until 1976 that the IOC and the IAAF Medical Commission decided to add anabolic steroids to the list of drugs for testing. It was in 1976, at the Montreal Olympics that there were eight positive tests for anabolic steroids.

Qualitative tests for testosterone were performed in 1982 followed by testing for human chorionic growth factor (HCG) and growth factor (GF) in 1985.

The above is only a very brief outline of the history of drugs and drug testing in sport. Does it matter? As a practicing doctor, the health and wellbeing of my patients is of paramount importance. The Hippocratic oath states that

'I will use those dietary regimens which will benefit my patients according to my greatest ability and judgement and I will do no harm or injustice to them'

So why test? Testing is there to deter not only athletes but also coaches and physicians in using any drugs on the current list of prohibited substances or methods. It is there to catch athletes and any others encouraging the athlete, actively involved in the use of drugs. From the physician's point of view it is there to educate and remind the athlete and any support staff of the potential harm both immediate and long term to his or her health following the use of such substances. We also have a role to remind them of the principle of 'fair play', a principle forgotten by a few high profile athletes but still maintained by the vast majority. Arthur Ashe, the Wimbledon tennis champion

'You've got to get to a stage in life where going for it is more important than winning of losing'

National Governing Bodies (NGB) or UK Anti-Doping now nominates individuals for inclusion in the National Registered Testing Pool (NRTP). Each athlete will be expected to provide up-to-date athletes 'Whereabouts Filings' [37] to ensure that the can be tested at anytime and anywhere with no advance notice. The athlete is expected to provide the following information:

- One hour slot every day
- Address of daily residence
- Regular activities (training, work etc)
- Competition schedule

Those athletes involved in team sports may be able to delegate this task to their coach, club or NGB. The rugby union teams that I am involved with full understand that each player is ultimately responsible for ensuring that the information given is accurate and complete, reaffirming the principle of strict liability. Further information can be obtained on the ADAMS web-site www.myadams.co.uk.

Athletes who are on the WADA 'whereabouts' list have presented in a similar fashion but are more likely to present to the sports physician via the National Governing Body (NGB) following a positive drug test. But positive drug test for anabolic steroids is declining in the athletic population as a whole in recent years according to data from UK Sport and WADA. Below are the numbers of test carried out in all sports and in selected sports that are of interest to the author during the period 2007 - 2010:

2007-2008

	In competition %	Out-of competition % 5	Total No	Elevated T/E ratio Cases to answer	Excluding elevated T/E ratio Cases to answer
All sports	38%	62%	7093	1	0
English FA	545	1038	1583	0	0
RFU	137(33%)	275(67%)	412	0	0
SRU	62(24%)	192(76%)	254	0	0
WRU	80(36%)	141(64%)	221	0	0
B/ building	23(100%)	0(0%)	23	0	0
W/lifting	38(34%)	75(66%)	113	0	0

FA = Football Association. IRB = International Rugby Board. RFU = Rugby Football Union. SRU = Scottish Rugby Union. WRU = Welsh Rugby Union. B/Building = body building. W/Lifting = weightlifting. T/E ratio = testosterone/epitestosterone ratio. Data from UKAD.

2008-2009

	In competition %	Out-of competition % 5	Total No	Elevated T/E ratio Cases to answer	Excluding elevated T/E ratio Cases to answer
All sports	38%	62%	7545	1	4
English FA	484	1129	1613	0	0
RFU	153(31%)	335(69%)	488	0	0
SRU	48(22%)	167(78%)	215	0	0
WRU	62(26%)	180(74%)	242	1	0
B/building	No data	No data	No data	No data	No data
W/lifting	37(41%)	53(59%)	90	0	0

FA = Football Association. IRB = International Rugby Board. RFU = Rugby Football Union. SRU = Scottish Rugby Union. WRU = Welsh Rugby Union. B/Building = body building. W/Lifting = weightlifting. T/E ratio = testosterone/epitestosterone ratio. Data from UKAD.

2009 – 2010

	In competition %	Out-of competition % 5	Total No	Elevated T/E ratio Cases to answer	Excluding elevated T/E ratio Cases to answer
All sports	39%	61%	7550	0	3
English FA	448(31%)	976(69%)	1424	0	0
RFU	152(26%)	441(74%)	593	0	0
SRU	60(24%)	188(76%	248	0	0
WRU	84(25%)	255(75%)	339	0	0
B/building	No data	No data	No data	No data	No data
W/lifting	37(46%)	44(54%)	81	0	0

FA = Football Association. IRB = International Rugby Board. RFU = Rugby Football Union. SRU = Scottish Rugby Union. WRU = Welsh Rugby Union. B/Building = body building. W/Lifting = weightlifting. T/E ratio = testosterone/epitestosterone ratio. Data from UKAD.

The World Anti Doping Association (WADA) make it abundantly clear that it is the athlete responsibility if a substance(s), or related substance(s), is/are found in a sample tested in or out of competition. The sports physician's first thoughts when faced with an athlete presenting with a positive test are:

1. Has the athlete taken a substance with the intent of cheating
2. Has the athlete inadvertently taken the substance as a simple remedy for a simple medical condition e.g. the common cold
3. Or none of the above and the test result is a false positive one?

Substances bought over-the counter for simple remedies are often stimulant drugs and glucocorticoids and some may be taken with the full knowledge that they are on the banned list. In such a case, this would be deemed to be a clear intent to 'cheat'. The use of anabolic steroids in the athletic population also demonstrates a clear attempt to gain unfair advantage but false positive test however can occur.

Exogenous anabolic steroids include:

17α-alkyl ester: stanozolol, methandienone, methyltestosterone, oxandrolone, oxymesterone

17β-OH ester: bolenone, methenolone, trenbolone, drostanolone, nandrolone

Endogenous anabolic steroids include:

androstenediol, androstenedione, dehydroepiandrosterone, dihydrotestosterone, testosterone and related substances

Testing involves identifying the drug or its metabolite however a specific
cut-off point for testosterone is difficult because of the large variation between
individuals. In 1983 the IOC adopted the testosterone to epitestosterone ratio
(T/E ratio) with an upper limit of 6 as evidence of exogenous testosterone use
or of a pathological condition. In 2004 this ratio was reduced to 4 by WADA
to reduce the number of false positives [38]. Testing is part of day-to-day life
in elite athletes but still does not seem to deter some athletes from anabolic
steroid use. The publicity surrounding the use of (and positive testing for)
anabolic steroids, might reinforce the belief in the general public and
recreational athlete that they are performance enhancing. Testing these groups
of individuals however is impractical

A positive test for nandrolone has been a topic of interest for some time.
Its main metabolites, namely 19-noradrosterone and 19-epiandrosterone and
19-noretiocholanolone, 19-norandrosterone are the most usual metabolite in
urine [39]. The IOC, in 1996 stated that a doping offence will be deemed to
have occurred if the urine concentration of 19-norandrosterone exceeds 2
ng/ml in men and curiously 5 ng/ml in women. Why there is a greater
concentration in women is difficult to understand. In 1982, Bjorkhem and Ek
[40] detected 19-norandrosterone in the urine of athletes who claimed never to
have used nandrolone.

Tests for the detection of 19- norandroserone have become more sensitive
over the years. A paper by Galan Martin [41] in 2001 found high levels of 19-
norandrosterone in five sportspeople with a range of between 4ng/ml and 14
ng/ml. One postmenopausal woman had a concentration of 19-norandrosteone
of 22 ng/ml. However there was no comment or further investigations to
explain the high levels seen in some of these individuals. It is well recognised
that there is a wide variation in the level of testosterone among males [42]. It is
therefore not unreasonable to assume that there could be a genetically
determined similar large variation in 19-norandrosterone. Exercise itself could
result in higher levels. High intensity exercise can increase the levels of
testosteroneandrostenedione and dehydroepiandrosterone due to increased
testicular production [43]. The mechanism however is not fully explained.

Supplementation with protein and carbohydrate drinks is commonplace in
my experience and contamination has always been a major concern. Athletes

often take additional minerals over the counter despite repeated warnings of the potential risk of contamination. Supplementation with zinc has been associated with an elevation in serum testosterone. Some authors have speculated that if supplementation with zinc is combined with intense exercise could result in increased levels of 19-norandrosterone, as the metabolism of 19-norstreoid may be similar to the metabolism of testosterone. Brilla [44] and his colleagues published a paper in 2000 when 30 mg of zinc (with magnesium) was given to football players every night for eight weeks. This resulted in a 33% increase the serum bound testosterone.

Tscholl [45] and his colleagues looked at the use of nutritional supplements and other medications during the FIFA World Cups in 2002 and 2006. 43% of players reported the use of supplements during the whole tournament in 2002 and 2006. Per match 31% and 35% used supplement in 2002 and 2006 respectively. In previous studies [46] coaches have been found to have a greater influence than doctors or sport dieticians. If so, this would result in a considerable amount of bias on the reported intake reported by team doctors. In my experience, conditioning coaches have the greatest influence in rugby union. In general, nutritional supplementation is not considered necessary in athletes with an adequate diet. However supplements can be useful in certain circumstance e.g. foreign travel when food intake can be erratic and choices can be restricted. In January 2011 the International Olympic Committee (IOC) published a consensus statement [47]:

> 'Athletes contemplating the use of supplements and sports foods should consider their efficacy, their cost, the risk to health and performanceand the potential for a positive doping test'

Is there a risk of a false positive in contact sport as a result of direct trauma to muscle? The *Cape Times* [48] reported an international rugby player testing positive for nandrolone at a level in breach of the WADA regulations (>2 ng/ml) having provided a sample after an intensely physical match. Could hypoglycaemic stress with is associated elevation in cortisol, glucagon and growth hormone have an effect. Cortisol levels rise in response to adrenocorticotrophic hormone which in itself increases adrenal androgens and hence an increase in urine 19-norandrosterone. This poses an interesting area for on-going research.

Is it time for the Sport Governing bodies or possibly the athlete to develop a steroid profile? A biological passport has been suggested which could contain retrospective data and the results of all endocrine investigations. This would overcome the issue of biological variability and give the athlete the assurance of a 'level playing field'. There are some ethical, legal and issues regarding cost to be address before this could be implemented.

Limited retrospective electronic data is available to the general practitioner, which would not be helpful in the event of a positive drug test but could be of value to identify adverse effects. It is my experience that the recreational user will have contacted the general practitioner with various medical conditions in the past, which might have been investigated. Such investigations might well have included a full blood count, haematocrit, liver function test, renal function test and even testosterone, follicle stimulating hormone and luteinising hormone levels. A biological passport would certainly be one way of protecting the innocent, educate and deter the user.

REFERENCES

[1]   Todd, T. Anabolic Steroids. The gremlins of Sport. *J Sports History* 1987;14:87-101.

[2]   Grogan, S. (1999) *Body image: understanding boy dissatisfaction in men, women and children.* London: Routledge.

[3]   Choi, P.Y.L., Pope, Jnr H.G., Olivardia, R. Muscle dysmorphia: a new syndrome in weightlifters. *Brit J Sports Med* 2002:36:375-377.

[4]   Buckley, W.E., Yesalis, C.E., Friedl, K., Anderson, W.A., Streit, A.L., Wright J. Estimated prevalence of anabolic steroids use among male high school seniors. *JAMA* 1988;260:3441-5.

[5]   Windsor, R., & Dumitru, D. Prevelence of anabolic steroid use by male and female adolescents. *Med Sci Sport Exerc* 1989:21(5):494-7.

[6]   Williamson, D.J. Anabolic steroid use among students at a British college of technology. *Brit J Sports Med* 1993;27(3):200-201.

[7]   The Advisory Council on Misuse of Drugs (ACMD). Consideration of the Anabolic Steroids. September 2010.

[8]   Harmer, P.A. Anabolic-androgenic steroid use among young male and female athletes: is the game to blame? *Brit J Sports Med* 2010;44:26-31.

[9]   Korkia, P.K., & Stimson, G.C. (1993) Anabolic steroid use in Great Britain; exploratory investigation. The Centre for Research on Drugs and health Behaviour. A report for the Department of Health, the Welsh Office and the Chief Scientist Office, Scottish Home and Health Department.

[10] Urhausen, A., Kindermann, W. Are the cardiac effects of anabolic steroid abuse in strength athletes reversible? *Heart* 2004;90:496-501.

[11] D'Andrea, A., Caso, P., Salerno, G., *et al.* Left ventricular early myocardial dysfunction after chronic misuse of anabolic androgenic steroids: Doppler myocardial and strain imaging analysis. *Br J Sports Med* 2007;41(3):149-55.

[12] Malarkey, W.B., Strauss, R.H., Leizman, D.J., Liggett, M., Demers, L.M. Endocrine effects in female weighlifters who self-administer testosterone and anabolic steroids. Am J Obstet Gynaecol 1991;165:1385-1390.

[13] Nygard, O, Nordrehaug, J.E. et al. Plasma homocysteine levels and mortality in patients with coronary artery disease. N Eng J Med 1997;337:230-6.

[14] Graham, M.R., Grace, F.M., Boobier, W., Hullin, D., *et al.* Homocysteine induced cardiovascular events: a consequence of long term anabolic-androgenic steroid (ASS) abuse. *Br J Sports Med* 2006; 40:644-648.

[15] Rosengren, A., Wilhelmsen, L., Eriksson, E., *et al.* Lipoprotein (a) and coronary heart disease: a prospective case-control study in a general population sample of middle aged men. *BMJ* 1990;301:1248-51.

[16] Hartgens, F., Rietjens, G., Keizer, H.A., Kuipers, H., Wolffenbuttel, B.H. Effects of androgenic-anabolic steroids on apolipoproteins and lipoprotein (a). *Brit J Sports Med* 2004;38:253-259.

[17] Krishnan P.V., Feng, Z.Z., Gordon, S.C. Prolonged intrahepatic cholestasis and renal failure secondary to anabolic steroid-enriched dietary supplements. *J Clin Gastroenterol* 2009;43(7):672-5.

[18] Socas, L., Zumbado, M., Perez-Luzardo O, Ramos, A., Perez, C., et al. Hepatocellular adenomas associated with anabolic androgenic steroid abuse in bodybuilders: a report of two cases and a review of the literature. *Brit J Sports Med* 2005;39:e27.

[19] Gorayski, P., Thompson, C.H., Subhash, H.S., Thomas, A.C. Hepatocellular carcinoma associated with recreational anabolic steroid use. *Brit J Sports Med* 2008;42:74-75.

[20] Daher, E.F., Silva Junior. G.B., Queiroz, A.L., Ramos, L.M., et al. Acute kidney injury due to anabolic steroid and vitamin supplement abuse: report of two cases and a literature review. *Int J Urol Nephrol* 2009;41(3):717-23.

[21] Kiraly, C.L., Alen, M., Korvola, J., Horsmanheimo, M. The effects of testosterone and anabolic steroids on the skin surface lipids and the

population of Propionibacteria acnes (P acnes) in young postpubertal men. *Acta Derm Venereol* 1968;68(1):21-6.

[22] Scott, M.J. 3rd, Scott AM. Effects of anabolic-androgenic steroids on the pilosebaceous unit. *Cutis* 1992;50(2):113-6.

[23] Rich, J.D., Foisie, C.K., Towe, C.W., Dickinson, P., McKenzie, M., Salas, C.M. Needle exchange program participation by anabolic steroid injectors. United Stares Drug and Alcohol Dependence 1998;56(2):157-60.

[24] Bahia, H., Platt, A., Hart, N.B., Bagulety, P. Anabolic steroid accelerated multicompartment syndrome following trauma. *Brit J Sport Med* 2000;34(4):308-309.

[25] Michna, H., Stangvos, C. The predisposition to tendon rupture after doping with anabolic steroids. *Int J sports Med* 1983;4:59S.

[26] Kramhoft, M., & Solgaard, S. Spontaneous rupture of the extensor polis longus tendon after anabolic steroids. *J Hand Surg* 1986;11:87.

[27] Freeman, B.J.C, & Rooker, G.D. Spontaneous rupture of the anterior cruciate ligament after anabolic stroids. *Brit J Sport Med* 1995;29(4)

[28] Liow R.Y.L, & Tavares, S. Bilateral rupture of the quadriceps tendon associated with anabolic steroids. *Brit J Sports Med* 1995;29(2):77-79.

[29] Cooper, C.J., Noakes, T.D., Dunne, T., Lambert, M.I., Rochford, K. A high prevalence of abnormal users of anabolic-androgenic steroids. *Brit J Sports Med* 1996;30:246-250.

[30] Greenway, P., & Greenway, M. General practitioner knowledge of prohibited substances in sport. *Brit J Sports Med* 1997;31:129-131.

[31] Marshall, E. The drug of champions. *Science* 1998;242:183-184.

[32] General medical Council (2004). Confidentiality: protecting and providing information. *http://gmc-uk.org/guidance*.

[33] The British Olympic Association's position statement on athlete confidentiality. *Brit J Sports Med* 2000;34:71-72 doi:10.1136/bjsm.34.1.71

[34] General Medical Council (2004). Confidentiality: protecting and providing information. *http://www.gmc-uk.org/guidance*.

[35] McNamee, M., & Phillips, N. Confidentiality, disclosure and doping in sports medicine. *Brit J Sports Med* 2011;45:174-177.

[36] Sperryn, P.N. 'Ethics in Sports Medicine – The Sports Physician' *Brit J Sports Med* 1980;14(2&3):84-89.

[37] *www.ukad.org.uk/pages/athletes*

[38] WADA Technical Document (TD2004EAAS): *Reporting and Evaluation Guidance for Testosterone, Epitestosterone, T/E ratio and Other Endogenous Steriods;* Montreal 2004. *http://www.wada-ama.org*

[39] Ozer, D., & Temizer, A. The determination of nanadrolone and its metabolites in the urine by gas chromatography-mass spectrometry. *Eur J Drug Metab Pharm*1997;22:421-5.

[40] Bjorkhem, E., & Ek, H. Detection and quantitation of 19-norandrosterone in urine by isotope dilution-mass spectrometry. *J Steriod Biochem Mol Biol* 1982;17:447-51.

[41] Galan Matin, A.M, Maynar Matino, J.l., Garcia de Tiedra, M.P. et al. Determination of nandrolone metabolites in urine samples from sedentary persons and sportsmen. *J Chromat B Biomed Sci Appl* 2001;761:229-36.

[42] Ganong, W.F. *Review of medical physiology.* Lange Medical Books, 1999;17:283; 19:345-60.

[43] Cumming, D., Brunsting, L., Strich, G. et al. Reproductive hormone increase in response to acute exercise in men. *Med Sci Sports Exerc* 1986;18:369-73

[44] Brilla, L.R., Conte, V. Effect of novel zinc-magnesium formulation on hormone and strength. *J Ex Physiol* 2000;3:26-36.

[45] Tscholl, P., Junge, A., Dvorak, J. The use of medication and nutritional supplements during FIFA World Cups 2002 and 2006. *Brit J Sport Med* 2008:42:725-730.

[46] Waddington, I., Malcolm, D., Roderick, M. et al. Drug use in English professional football. *Brit J Sport Med* 2005:39(4):e18.

[47] *http://www.olympic.org/Documents/Reports/EN/CONSENSUS-FINAL-v8-en.pdf*

[48] Nel, S. Springbok rugby player tests positive for steroids. *Cape Times* 2000;Nov 3:26.

In: Perspectives on Anabolic Androgenic ....   ISBN: 978-1-62081-243-3
Editors: F. Grace and J. S. Baker   © 2012 Nova Science Publishers, Inc.

Chapter 4

THE EFFECTS OF NON-THERAPEUTIC ANABOLIC ANDROGENIC STEROID (AAS) USE ON CARDIAC STRUCTURE AND FUNCTION

Fergal M. Grace[*,1], *Nick Sculthorpe*[2], *Julien S. Baker*[1] *and Lon Kilgore*[1]

[1] Department Sport & Exercise Sciences, University of the West of Scotland, Hamilton, South Lanarkshire, Scotland, UK
[2] Department of Sport & Exercise Sciences, University of Bedfordshire, Bedford, England, UK

FOREWORD

There has long been a call in medical and sports medicine literature for information pertaining to the long-term use of high dose AAS as used by weightlifters and bodybuilders. However, this is particularly challenging for researchers as such users take many times the therapeutic dose and no ethical board would possibly approve a study whereby participants receive high dose AAS. The best that can currently be achieved in studies involving human

* Address for correspondence: Dr. Fergal Grace, Senior Lecturer in Sport, Health & Exercise, University of the West of Scotland, Hamilton, South Lanarkshire, Scotland, ML3 OJB, United Kingdom. Tel: 01698 898271 ext: 8508, e-mail: fergal.grace@uws.ac.uk.

subjects is to recruit individuals who have habitually taken AAS in supra-physiological doses for a number of successive years. There is also an inherent issue of quality control, as non-therapeutic AAS users often take other drugs, whether recreational or performance enhancing, which can confound study data. Further, AAS users obtain their drugs from black market sources that are completely unregulated and products may contain /no other active ingredient (See Chapter One for further discussion).

AAS studies should confirm drug use through urinalysis and indentify active ingredients where possible. However, this is only achievable in a minority of cases and it should not dissuade researchers from obtaining and publishing data on case studies of cardiovascular consequences associated with AAS use as they are almost certainly underrepresented in the medical literature.

ABSTRACT

Studies investigating the effects of Anabolic Androgenic Steroids (AAS) on the cardiovascular system have been present in the medical literature over the past forty years. The present chapter reviews the available literature on the impact that AAS use has on cardiovascular structure and function from the more popular studies in the 1980s, investigating the effects of AAS on cholesterol levels to the more currently popular studies that aim to identify the underlying mechanisms behind remodeling of cardiac muscle. There is currently good progress being made in understanding the physiological mechanisms behind AAS induced cardio-toxicity from both the in vitro and animal model. If current rates of progress are continued and the medical research community continues to publish both controlled and case studies then a clearer understanding of the mechanisms behind cardiovascular problems resulting from AAS use are expected in the near future.

I. AAS IN BLOOD LIPIDS AND LIPOPROTEINS

In the 1980s, both media and medical interest in cholesterol as a risk factor for coronary heart disease coincided with the relatively new topic of anabolic androgenic steroid (AAS) use. Studies combining both areas of medical interest identified unfavourable effects of AAS on blood cholesterol profiles [1,2,3] and there was a simultaneous upsurge in the medical literature outlining these effects [4,5]. In the late 1970s, data from the Framingham Study identified that depressed HDL-Cholesterol (HDL-C) were significantly and independently associated with an increased coronary risk [6]. This was confirmed by further analyses based on longer follow up [7,8]. Subsequent cohort studies confirmed this association between low HDL-C and elevated Low Density Lipoprotein (LDL-C) on adverse coronary [9] and cerebro-vascular outcomes [10].

In the mid 1980s, the majority of AAS related studies employed either cross sectional or prospective design examining weightlifters/bodybuilders self-administering large doses of two or more AAS. The extremity of negative blood lipid alterations induced by AAS's has been described as being more profound than any pharmacological [4,5,11] or non-pharmacological [4] agents to date. A minority of studies at this time [2,3,4,5] utilised a controlled therapeutic dose. Such studies favoured the more convenient, therapeutic doses of 17--alkylated AAS rather than Parenteral (injectable) AAS.

The following two decades saw a multitude of AAS studies confirming these initial findings The majority of studies were of prospective or cross-sectional design examining weightlifters/bodybuilders and recreational gym users self-administering large doses of two or more AAS [12,18]. A minority of studies [2,3,19,20] have utilised a controlled therapeutic dose. Such early studies favoured the more convenient, therapeutic doses of oral (17--alkylated) AAS rather than Parenteral AAS. In the early 1990s, with the implementation of World Health Organisation task force investigation on the effectiveness of AAS as contraceptives, therapeutic interest centered around the injectable esterified AAS; *Testosterone Enanthate*. A meta-analysis [21] has reviewed the effects of such testosterone esters on blood lipids in hypogonadal men. This meta-analysis reviewed 20 studies of therapeutic AAS administration (1987-1999), and reported a small dose dependent decrease in HDL-C (mean 11%) and concomitant declines in total cholesterol and increases LDL-C (mean 9%). The importance of this review is that it identified that lipid-altering effects of AAS were more profound when 17--alkylated drugs were used.

The lack of a dose relationship in oral AAS studies was further identified in an elegant and often quoted review [22] outlining the impact of AAS Lipid sub-fractions in fifteen studies. This review identified a weighted average decrement of 52% in HDL in fifteen prospective cohort studies and 51% in cross-sectional studies with increases in LDL in the region of 36%. It further identified that the decrement in HDL was more pronounced on HDL2, which was shown to be reduced by an average of 78%. Depressions in HDL3 were reported to be less uniform and dramatic than those of HDL2 and total HDL-C concentrations. The specific targeting of the HDL2 subfraction is considered to be due to the effect of the enzyme Hepatic Triglyceride Lipase (HTGL) which has a particular affinity to bind and catabolise HDL and particularly the HDL2 subfraction through its phospholipase activity [22]. Evidence of the phospholipic activity of HTGL has been idenfied in some of the earlier therapeutic AAS dose studies [2,3,19] and further evidenced in studies where participants used two or more AAS in supraphysiological doses of AAS [23,26].

It has also been identified that the deleterious effects of AAS on blood lipids and Apolipoproteins is transient. The available literature investigating this particular aspect would suggest that HDL-C levels begin to decrease immediately after AAS consumption [20, 22] that they reach their trough between 1 and 4 weeks after initiating AAS use [2, 20,27] and return to pre-treatment concentrations following 3 to 5 weeks [28,29,30], 6 weeks [14] and within 3 months [31] following cessation of use. Two AAS related studies have suggesting that recovery of blood lipids following AAS administration may take longer than three months [17,26], though, though one of these failed to report any hormonal levels.

Apolipoprotein A-1 (Apo A-1), the major Apoprotein of HDL and to a lesser extent Apolipoproein A-II (Apo A-II) have also shown to follow a similar reduction to that of HDL following therapeutic doses [1,2,5,27] and supraphysiological doses of AAS [13,24,32,33,34]. Studies similarly reporting on the effect of AAS on LDL and its major Apolipoprotein (Apo-B) consistently report elevations in serum values much the same as increases in HDL though its effects are less dramatic [2-3,5,13-15,19,21-22,28,31,33-34]. Again, the 17--alkylated AAS are associated with producing a more profound deleterious effect on Apoliproteins [20,22,33,36]. The monitoring of Total Cholestorol (Tot-C) is somewhat superfluous. Although there is a marked increased Atherogenic profile as androgen induced increases in LDL are offset by the decreased HDL resulting in no overall change in Tot-C.

The transitory effect of AAS on blood lipids and Apolipoproteins makes it difficult to ascertain the long term Atherogenic risk from the use of these drugs. In relation to this, the majority of AAS users use AAS intermittently in a process known as 'Cycling' in the belief that this avoids developing a tolerance to a particular AAS drug and to minimise the potential side-effects associated with AAS use.

II. AAS ON SYSTEMIC BLOOD PRESSURE

Androgen induced hypertension tends to be one of the most frequent yet inconclusive health risks associated with AAS [39-40]. Available evidence on the blood pressure response to concomitant AAS use remains equivocal [13,41]. '

Some studies have reported AAS associated increases in blood pressure [22,42-43], while others have failed to demonstrate any effect of AAS on systemic blood pressure [44-46].

Discrepancies between studies may be due in part, to the low subject numbers traditionally used in AAS investigations. Rate pressure product (RPP), defined as a function of heart rate and systolic pressure provides an indirect indicator of cardiac output and hence myocardial oxygen demand has been identified to be elevated in amateur bodybuilders using AAS [43].

The action by which AAS may have caused cycle dependent increases in blood pressure in the AAS using group is unknown. It has been suggested elevated levels of 11- deoxycorticosterone may be responsible [47].

This implies a direct inhibition of the 11--Hydroxylation by the androgen resulting in a consequent overproduction of 11-deoxycorticosterone by the adrenal cortex', in a process similar to the apparent mineralocorticoid excess syndrome as seen in patients with Cushing's syndrome.

In addition, catecholamines may be involved in the activation of renin secretion, the increase in resting heart rate and -oxidation of adipose tissue. Androgens may also increase renal renin secretion [13].

This hypothesis may be further supported by the increased plasma aldosterone levels that have been identified in both human [48] and bovine model [49], potentially affecting arterial blood pressure through increases in cardiac output and total peripheral resistance.

The data from the available body of evidence are equivocal. There are those that support the assertion that AAS acutely influences blood pressure [22,42,51], specifically diastolic blood pressure [13].

However, many studies studies do no not support the hypothesis that AAS use causes hypertension [43,50-54].

There is some evidence that AAS use increases cardiovascular strain via increases in blood pressure at rest [43] which is exaggerated during acute exercise [55].

III. EFFECTS OF AAS ON VASCULAR ENDOTHELIAL FUNCTION

The relationship between the use of Anabolic Androgenic Steroids (AAS) and vascular function has received some attention over the past decade. There is some evidence of improved vascular function when therapeutic doses of testosterone are used [56].

Owing to both the relatively recent medical application of required expertise and expense associated with the technique, there is considerably less scientific investigation on vascular health than the traditionally popular investigations on blood lipids, blood pressure and echocardiographic studies. However, owing to the progressive nature of atherosclerosis, and the key influence of endothelial dysfunction on atherosclerotic disease progression such studies are important to establish risk in the AAS user.

The potential for AAS to dramatically affect endothelial vasodilatory response to nitric oxide mediated dilatory function was identified as early as 1993 [57] where an AAS using subject was identified as an outlier in a study examining endothelial response to methacholine and sodium nitroprusside. Vasodilatory response subsequently returned to normal following a period of abstinence from AAS use.

Flow medidated dilatation (FMD) is a relatively new non-invasive method used to assess arterial function with abnormal values being linked to future cardiovascular events [58]. Two studies in 2001 identified an altered flow mediated dilatation in response to glyceryl trinitrite (GTN) in AAS using bodybuilders [59-60] suggestive of the potential for AAS to affect vascular smooth muscle function. A further progressive study conducted by Lane and colleagues conducted at the Cardiff medical school in Wales, UK, found an impaired endothelial-independent dilatation in both current AAS users and those that had been abstinent for a period greater than three months [54]. Given that two of the three studies showing a reduced FMD in these AAS related studies [54,59]. Although there are some similar findings in non-AAS related studies [61-62] it remains to be elucidated if prolonged continuous resistance training associated with bodybuilding exercise can negatively affect vascular function.

It has been suggested that AAS may have a directly negative effect on the vascular endothelium through a direct effect on the nitric oxide dilatory system [63] which in turn increases arterial stiffness and reduces FMD. AAS have been also shown to retard endothelial growth [64].

There is a further existing hypothesis that AAS may magnify the effects of certain vasoconstrictors [65], however an increase in the adhesion of monocytes to endothelial cells has been demonstrated [66] via an up-regulation of vascular cell adhesion molecule-1 (VCAM-1) in an in vitro model. Further in vitro research has identified Testosterone also induces apoptosis of endothelial cells in vitro and promotes proliferation and migration of vascular smooth muscle cells, which are known to contribute to the development of atherosclerotic lesions [67]. Indeed, although first suggested from in vitro work [68], there is a growing body of recent evidence that AAS directly contribute to coronary lesions in the animal model [67,69].

Homocysteine (HCY), a thiol containing amino acid formed from the intracellular demethylation of methionine, at elevated levels, is considered to be an independent marker of endothelial damage and consequently cardiovascular risk [70]. Although Zmuda and colleagues (1997) did not find any effect of AAS on HCY concentrations [71], a more recent study [35] identified elevated HCY in both (long term) current AAS users and users that had been abstinent for 3 months, highlighting that AAS may induce endothelial risk, which may persist months following withdrawal. In addition to HCY, C-Reactive Protein (CRP), another independent cardiovascular risk factor through a direct effect on vascular endothelium [72] has been shown to be elevated in AAS users in tow studies comparing AAS users with control bodybuilders and sedentary controls [73-74].

Although there is a sound evidence to suggest that the use of AAS, particularly in supraphysiological doses may produce serious consequences on vascular endothelium. Further investigative work is necessary to identify whether altered endothelial function is as a result of bodybuilding exercise or whether the combination of bodybuilding exercise and AAS consumption produces a negatively additive effect.

IV. AAS ON HAEMOSTATIC SYSTEM

Although there is little direct evidence that AAS directly affect the haemostatic system, there is an ever-growing database of case reports in the medical literature highlighting serious thrombolytic cardiovascular complications including hypertension, cardiomyopathy, stroke, pulmonary embolism, fatal and nonfatal arrhythmias, and myocardial infarction have been reported with supraphysiologic doses of anabolic androgenic steroids (AAS).

Much of our knowledge for the potential for AAS to affect blood volume, platelet aggregation and the coagulation cascade come from studies investigating therapeutic applications of AAS in the 1970s and 1980s. Some of the earliest studies lend support to the suggestion that AAS had therapeutic potential through an activation of the fibrinolytic system [75-77]. Increases in erythropoietic activity was evidences through consistent elevations of hemoglobin was an almost universally consistent finding [78] In therapeutic studies, Hemoglobin is shown to increase by approximately 10% [79] and even in therapeutic doses are associated with the development of polycythemia [80-81] in a dose dependent fashion [82-83]. 17-∂-alkylated (oral) AAS were shown to increase plasminogen activator activity and antithrombin III in a number of studies in mid-1980's [84-85]. As the clinical effects of AAS were inconsistent and ultimately disappointing [86,87], there was a large decline in AAS related investigations on the haemostatic system by the beginning of the 1990s.

Ferenchick (1991) first identified the connection between AAS and the potential to develop thrombolytic disease in a weightlifting population [88]. The following year Ferenchick and colleagues identified a potential trend towards increased platelet counts and platelet aggregation in 28 weightlifters [89] in the absence of a control group for comparison. Further study in a group of bodybuilders showed that AAS may cause a hypercoagulable state [90] by an increase in production of thromboxane A_2 and platelet thromboxane A_2 receptor density as well as aggregation responses and a decrease in production of prostaglandins [91].

The first carefully controlled study to report a connection between AAS and potential thrombosis resulting from non-therapeutic use was reported by Ferenchick et al. (1995) in a group of weightlifters abusing AAS [92]. The authors concluded that the supraphysiological doses of AAS used by some of the weightlifters accelerated activation of their hemostatic systems evidenced by increases in both thrombin and plasmin, which could potentially result in vascular occlusion. Although there is limited direct evidence that AAS are prothrombotic when used in a non-therapeutic manner, therapeutic studies provide useful and important clues on the identification of pathogenesis. One of the rare recently controlled studies [93] using a replacement dose of an oral AAS (20mg oxandrolone/day over 14 days) reported an activation of the fibrinolytic system thorough a decrease in plasminogen activator inhibitor (PAI-1) following short term use.

Unfortunately, the data on the use of supraphysiological doses of AAS in humans are mainly offered as case reports or small studies that lack adequate control groups [94]. In addition, the data available in the literature does not account for the steroid type(s) or dose, as neither may be known. In addition, AAS users presenting as clinical cases for emergency treatment may also be taking concomitant stimulants, such as ephedrine, which can confound data and the potential for adverse events. However, given that there is a recognized dose dependent influence of AAS on the haemostatic system [82,95-96] and the few available studies in weight lifters and bodybuilders show both pro-coagulatory and fibrinolytic activation. Indeed, sudden death and acute embolytic events may represent under appreciated risks of AAS use and are thought to be under represented in the medical literature [97]. Such cases are vitally important in raising awareness on adverse consequences of AAS on the cardiovascular system.

The consequences of activating the haemostaic system are that systemic emboli may terminate in the brain, heart or lungs with potentially serious consequences. There are multiple case reports of systemic emboli and thrombotic complications occurring in AAS using athletes. Case reports of otherwise young healthy men presented with cerrebro-vascular accident [97-98] in the late 1980's. Since then there has been a steady increase in the number of case reports of acute thrombotic complications such as cerrebro-vascular accident (97-105), Pulmonary embolus [106-108], Acute coronary thrombus [109-118].

IV. AAS ON MYOCARDIAL STRUCTURE AND FUNCTION

Significant changes to myocardial structure resulting from AAS use with concomitant bodybuilding exercise were identified in the late 1980s. Both left ventricular (LV) mass and wall thickness in addtion to an increased septal wall thickness were identified and supported by early studies on AAS users [119-120] and when compared to non-AAS using controls. [121,124]. However, in keeping with most medical aspects associated with AAS use, studies are not completely consistent [123] which not helped by the many confounding variables that are beyond the control of the investigating scientist.

Fewer studies have shown AAS using participants to present with an increased LV cavity size without an increase in LV wall and septal wall thickness [124], more commonly associated with eccentric volume overload of athletes heart in distance runners rather than concentric pressure overload that has become synonymous with weight lifting exercises [121-122].

The more recent advent of tissue Doppler techniques has allowed for a more detailed investigation of cardiac dynamics. Studies that have examined functional cardiac dynamics through the measurement of mitral annular velocities have identified a lack of difference between AAS using bodybuilders, bodybuilding controls and sedentary controls [125] whereas others have found altered ejection fraction in AAS users [126] which may be partly explained if further evidence is found to support the in vitro work of LeGros and colleagues [68]. This work identified an up-regulation of Lysyl oxidase which is shown to be a key enzyme responsible for initiating cross-links between adjacent collagen molecules and may have an impact on myocardial collagen content.

The potential of diastolic funicition to be altered by the concentric hypertrophy associated with resistance exercise has received more attention. Diastolic filling velocity has been shown to be both unaffected in AAS using bodybuilders compared with controls [122,127] though the latter identified significant differences in early to late diastolic tissue velocities. Reduction in diastolic filling and relaxation time could be explained by a reduction in myocardial elasticity as identified by the work of LeGros. Further explanation for direct targeting of myocytes can be evidenced in two further studies that have shown that androgens may affect extracellular calcium mobilisation [128] and apoptosis of myocytes in the rat model [129].

ELECTROPHYSIOLOGY

Electrophysiological measurement can have some use in identifying myocardial alterations such as left ventricular hypertrophy (LVH), cardiovascular disease (CVD) on inhomogenous conduction through the myocardium, which may be perpetuated by AAS use. There have been some previous associations between atrial fibrillation considered to be induced by AAS administration [130-131]. Prolonged QT interval is a phenomenon that has been identified in athletes following endurance training and power lifting [132], However, androgen use has been shown to produce a shortening of QT [133] interval which is supported by evidence of altered potassium protein channel activity in the rabbit model [134].

Recently, the presence of late ventricular potentials (Lps) have been evidenced by a research group examining myocardial electrophysiology following prolonged. AAS use [135]. Lp's are high amplitude, low requency potentials located in the terminal portion of the QRS complex. The study by

Sculthorpe and colleagues [135] reported an increased presence of Lp's following functional diagnostic exercise testing in a group of current and previous AAS users. Lp's are considered to reflect an area of slow inhomogeneous or delayed tissue which may provide a reentry mechanism for malignant tachyarrhythmia. Such studies should be of particular concern to AAS users as it suggests a triggering mechanism for atrial fibrillation with the potential for sudden cardiac death.

Testosterone has been shown to interact directly with the NO system. Activation of this pathway induces shortening in the duration of the action potential by activating the slow component of delayed rectifier potassium current (Iks) and inhibiting L-type calcium currents [136-137]. Furthermore, animal studies have shown that androgens have the potential to interfere with potassium channel function [134,138] which adds to the recently growing evidence that AAS affect electrical function through the myocardium [133,135,139-140]. There is currently some good work being done in the animal model [141-142] and much of the future progress on identifying the underlying cardiovascular pathologies resulting from the combination of exercise and high-dose AAS as used by bodybuilders and weightlifters is likely to come from this emerging area.

One of the more serious adverse affect resulting from alteration to cardiac structure and function is that of myocardial infarction. Case reports of myocardial infarction associated with AAS use emerged in the late 1980s and have continued to date [144-156]. Cases of atrial fibrillation [157] hypertrophic cardiomyopathy [158,159,160] and myocarditis [112,118,160-161] have been also been identified.

Cases of sudden death associated with AAS are almost certainly under-reported in the medical literature. There have been some publication of cases/multiple cases where autopsy has been performed on former AAS users who died suddenly which reveal concentric hypertrophy, myocyte necrosis and dilated cardiomyopathy [161-166] as the likely causes of mortality. Post mortem cases suggest the potential for AAS to directly affect cardiac structure at both the cellular and functional level and that the combination of heavy resistance exercise with concomitant AAS use can produce pathological changes to myocardial structure. Overall mortality rates have been estimated as being 4.6 times higher in AAS users compared with controls [167] in a popularized post survey of former power-lifters, which examined mortality of 62 male powerlifters placed 1st-5th in weight series 82.5-125 kg in Finnish championships during 1977-1988. 12-year follow-up indicated 12.9% mortality for the powerlifters compared to 3.1% in the control population.

Although there were three cases of myocardial infarction, many of the mortality cases were non cardiac in origin.

The difficulty with case report studies is that AAS using patients presenting with acute cardiovascular problems may also be engaged in polypharmacy, using drugs such as amphetamines, cocaine or ephedra, each of which are associated with acute cardiac events [143]. This is possibly the single biggest factor that affects the defining link between AAS and coronary structure and function. As urinalysis is largely unavailable in the clinical situation, this remains a constant confounding factor in AAS research. Given that it is impossible to conduct studies where supraphysiological doses of AAS are administered to humans, we will be relying on further case studies in addition to carefully controlled monitoring studies to identify cardiovascular issues resulting from AAS use in humans. There are a number of ongoing studies in the animal model that are encouraging in identifying the underlying mechanisms of cardiac damage in humans [141-142].

REFERENCES

[1]   Cheung MC, Albers JJ, Wahl PW & Hazzard WR High density lipoproteins during hypolipidemic therapy. *Atherosclerosis*, 1980;35: 215-228.

[2]   Haffner, SM, Kushwaha RS, Foster DM, et al. Studies on the metabolic mechanism of reduced high density lipoproteins during anabolic steroid therapy. *Metabolism*, 1983;32: 413-420.

[3]   Glueck C. Nonpharmacologic and pharmacologic alteration of high-density lipoprotein cholesterol: Therapeutic approaches to prevention of atheroclerosis. *American Heart Journal*, 1985; 110: 1107-1115.

[4]   Thompson PD, Cullinane EM, Sady SP, et al. Contrasting effects of testosterone and stanozolol on serum lipoprotein levels. *Journal of the American Medical Association*, 1989;261: 1165-1168.

[5]   Gordon T, Castelli WP, Hjortland MC et al. High density lipoprotein as a protective factor against coronary heart disease. The Framingham Study. *Am J Med* 1977;62:707–714.

[6]   Wilson PW, Abbott RD, Castelli WP. High density lipoprotein cholesterol and mortality. The Framingham Heart Study. *Arteriosclerosis* 1988;8:737–741.

[7]   Castelli WP, Garrison RJ, Wilson PW et al. Incidence of coronary heart disease and lipoprotein cholesterol levels. The Framingham Study. *JAMA* 1986;256:2835–2838

[8]   Coldbourt U, Yaari S, Medalie JH. Isolated low HDL cholesterol as a risk factor for coronary heart disease mortality. A 21-year follow-up of 8000 men. *Arterioscler Thromb Vasc Biol* 1997;17:107–113.

[9]   Tanne D, Yaari S, Goldbourt U. High-density lipoprotein cholesterol and risk of ischemic stroke mortality. A 21-year follow-up of 8586 men from the Israeli Ischemic Heart Disease Study. *Stroke* 1997;28:83–87.

[10] Henkin, Y., Jackson, A.C., Oberman, A. Secondary dyslipidemia. Inadvertent effects of drugs in clinical practice. *Journal of the American Medical Association*, 1992;267: 961-968.

[11] Hurley BF, Seals DR, Hagberg JM, et al. High Density Lipoprotein cholesterol in bodybuilders v powerlifters. *Journal of the American Medical Association*, 1984; 252: 507-513.

[12] Fröhlich J, Kullmer T, Urhausen, A, et al. Lipid Profile of body builders with and without self-administration of anabolic steroids. *European Journal of Applied Physiology* 1989; 59: 98-103.

[13] Kuipers H, Wijnen JAG, Hartgens F. & Willems, SMM. Influence of anabolic steroids in body composition, blood pressure, lipid profile and liver functions in body builders. *International Journal of Sports Medicine*, 1991;12: 413-418.

[14] Hartgens F, Rietjiens G, Keizer HA, *et al.* Effects of androgenic-anabolic steroids on apolipoproteins and lipoprotein(a). *British Journal of Sports Medicine*, 2004;38 (3): 253-9.

[15] Palatini P, Giada F, Garavelli G, et al. Cardiovascular effects of anabolic steroids in weight-trained subjects. *Journal of Clinical Pharmacology*, 1996 36: 1132-1140.

[16] Urhausen A, Albers T, & Kindermann W. Reversibility of the effects on blood cells, lipids, liver function and hormones in former anabolic-androgenic steroid abusers. *J Steroid Biochem Mol Biol*, 2003;84, 2-3, Proceedings of the 15th International Symposium of the Journal of Steroid Biochemistry and Molecular Biology - Poster Presentations, February 2003, Pages 369-375

[17] Bonetti A, Tirelli F, Catapano A., et al (2008) Side effects of anabolic androgenic steroid use, *International Journal of Sports Medicine*, 29 (8):679-87

[18] Applebaum-Bowden D, Haffner SM, Hazzard WR. The dyslipoproteinemia of anabolic steroid therapy: Increase in hepatic

triglyceride lipase precedes the drop in high-density lipoprotein cholesterol. *Metabolism*, 1987; 36: 949-952.

[19] Thompson PD, Cullinane EM, Sady SP, et al. Contrasting effects of testosterone and stanozolol on serum lipoprotein levels. *Journal of the American Medical Association*, 1989;261: 1165-1168.

[20] Whitsel EA, Boyko, EJ, Matsumoto AM, et al. Intramuscular testosterone esters and plasma lipids in hypogonadal men: a meta-analysis. *American Journal of Medicine*, 2001;111(4): 261-269.

[21] Glazer G. Artherogenic Effects of Anabolic Steroids on Serum Lipid Levels. A Literature Review. *Archives of Internal Medicine*, 1991;151(10): 1925-1933.

[22] Lenders JWM, Demacker PNM, Vos, JA, et al. Deleterious effects of anabolic steroids on serum lipoproteins, blood pressure, and liver function in amateur body builders. *International Journal of Sports Medicine*, 1988;9: 19-23.

[23] Zuliani U, Bernardini B, Catapano A, et al. Effects of anabolic steroids, testosterone, and HGH on blood lipids and echocardiographic parameters in body builders. *International Journal of Sports Medicine*, 1988;10: 62-66

[24] Zmuda J, Fahrenbach M, Burrows T. et al. The effect of testosterone aromatization on high-density lipoprotein cholesterol level and postheparin lipolytic activity, *Metabolism*, 1993;42, (4), 446-450

[25] Kleiner SM, Calabrese LH, Fielder KM, et al. Dietary influences on cardiovascular disease risk in anabolic steroid-using and non-using bodybuilders. *Journal of the American College of Nutrition*, 1989;8: 109-119.

[26] Kiraly CL. Androgenic-anabolic steroid effects on serum and skin surface lipids, on red cells and on liver enzymes. *International Journal of Sports Medicine*, 1988;9: 249-252.

[27] Webb LO, Laskarzewski PM, Glueck PJ. Severe depression of high-density lipoprotein cholesterol levels in weightlifters and body builders by self-administered exogenous testosterone and anabolic-androgenic steroids. *Metabolism*, 1984;33: 971-975.

[28] Peterson GE, Fahey TD, HDL-C in five elite athletes using anabolic-androgenic steroids. *The Physician and Sports Medicine*, 1984;12: 1

[29] Costill DL, Pearson, DR, Fink WL. Anabolic steroid use among athletes: changes in HDL-C levels. *The Physician and Sports Medicine*, 1984;12: 113-117.

[30] Hartgens, F & Kuipers H. Effects of androgenic-anabolic steroids in athletes. *Sports Medicine*, 2004;34: (8): 513-554.

[31] Cohen LI, Hartford CG, Rogers GG. Lipoprotein(a) and cholesterol in bodybuilders using anabolic androgenic steroids. *Medicine and Science in Sports and Exercise*, 1996;28: 176-179.

[32] Friedl KE, Hannan CJ, Jones RE & Plymate SR. High-Density lipoprotein cholesterol is not decreased if an aromatizable androgen is administered. *Metabolism,* 1990;39(1): 69-74.

[33] Dickerman RD, McConcathy WJ, Zachariah NY. Testosterone, sex hormone-binding globulin, lipoproteins and vascular disease risk. *Journal of Cardiovascular Risk*, 1997;4: 363-367.

[34] Singh AB, Hsia S, Alaupovic P. (2002). The effects of varying doses of Testosterone on insulin sensitivity, plasma lipids, apolipoproteins, and C-reactive protein in healthy young men. *J Clin Endocrinol Metab*, 2002;87 (1): 136-143.

[35] Graham MR. Grace FM, Boobier W, et al. Homocystine induced cardiovascular events: a consequence of long term anabolic-androgenic steroid (AAS) abuse. *Br J Sports Med*; 2006;40:644-648.

[36] Grace FM, Baker JS, Davies B. Anabolic androgenic steroid use in recreational gym users: a regional sample of the Mid-Glamorgan area. *J Subst Use* 2001;6:189–95.

[37] Baginsky ML, Brown WV, A new method for the measurement of lipoprotein lipase in postheparin plasma using sodium dodecyl sulfate for the inactivation of hepatic triglyceride lipase. *J. Lipid Res.* 1979;20: 548–556.

[38] Blades B, Vega GL, Grundy SM. Activities of lipoprotein lipase and hepatic triglyceride lipase in postheparin plasma of patients with low concentrations of HDL cholesterol. *Arterioscler Thromb.* 1993;13: 1227–1235.

[39] Melchert RB & Welder AA. Cardiovascular effects of androgenic anabolic steroids. *Med Sci Sport Exerc* 1995; 27:1252-1262.

[40] Perry H, Littlepage B. Dying to be big: a review of anabolic steroid use. *BJSM* 1992: 4(26):259-261.

[41] Morrison CL. Cocaine misuse in anabolic steroid users. *J Perform Enhan Drug* 1996; 1(1):10-15.

[42] Friedl KE, Dettori JR, Hannan, CJ. et al. Comparison of the effects of high dose testosterone and 19-nortestosterone to a replacement dose of testosterone on strength and body composition in normal men. *J Steroid Biochem Mol Biol* 1991; 40:607-612.

[43] Grace F, Sculthorpe N, Baker J, Davies B. Blood pressure and rate pressureproduct response in males using high-dose anabolic androgenic steroids (AAS). *J Sci Med Sport*. 2003 Sep;6(3):307-12.

[44] Palatini P, Giada F, Garavelli G. et al. Cardiovascular effects of anabolic steroids in weight-trained subjects. *J Clin Pharmacol* 1996; 36:1132-40.

[45] Thompson PD, Sadaniantz A, Cullinane EM. et al. Left ventricular function is not impaired in weight-lifters who use anabolic steroids. *J Am Coll Cardiol* 1996: 19:278-82.

[46] De Piccoli B, Giada F, Benettin A. et al. Anabolic steroid use in bodybuilders: an echocardiographic study of left ventricle morphology and function. *Int J Sports Med* 1991; 12:408-12.

[47] Rockhold RW. Cardiovascular toxicity of anabolic steroids. *Ann Rev Pharmacol Toxicol* 1993; 33:497-520.

[48] Christowski K, Kozera J, Grucza R. Medical consequences of anabolic steroid abuse. *Biol Sport* 2000; 17:134-152.

[49] Beutel A, Bergamaschi CT, Campos RR. Effects of chronic anabolic steroid treatment on tonic and reflex cardiovascular control in male rats. *J Steroid Biochem Mol Biol* 2005; 93: 43-48.

[50] Hartgens F, Van Marken Lichtenbelt WD, Ebbing S. et al. Body composition and anthropometry in bodybuilders: regional changes due to nandrolone decanoate administration. *Int J Sports Med* 2001; 22(3):235-241.

[51] Messerli FH & Fröhlich ED. High blood pressure: A side effect of drugs, poisons, and food. *Arch Intern Med* 1979; 139: 682-687.

[52] Urhausen A, Albers T, Kindermann W. Are the cardiac effects of anabolic steroid abuse in strength athletes reversible? *Heart* 2004; 90:496-501.

[53] Kawano H, Tanimoto M, Yamamoto K, Sanada K, Gando Y, Tabata I, et al. Resistance training in men is associated with increased arterial stiffness and blood pressure but does not adversely affect endothelial function as measured by arterial reactivity to the cold pressor test. *Exp Physiol*. 2008 Feb;93(2):296-302.

[54] Lane HA, Grace F, Smith JC, Morris K, Cockcroft J, Scanlon MF, et al. Impaired vasoreactivity in bodybuilders using androgenic anabolic steroids. *Eur J Clin Invest*. 2006Jul;36(7):483-8.

[55] Riebe D, Fernhall B, Thompson PD. The blood pressure response to exercise in anabolic steroid users. *Med Sci Sports Exerc*. 1992 Jun;24(6):633-7.

[56] Ong PJ, Patrizi G, Chong WC, et al. Testosterone enhances flow-mediated brachial artery reactivity in men with coronary artery disease. *Am J Cardiol.* 2000 Jan 15;85(2):269-72.

[57] Green DJ, Cable NT, Rankin JM, et al. Anabolic steroids and vascular responses. *Lancet.* 1993;342(8875):863.

[58] Gokce N, Keaney JF, Hunter LM, et al. Predictive value of noninvasively determined endothelial dysfunction for long-term cardiovascular events in patients with peripheral vascular disease. *J Am Coll Cardiol.* 2003 May 21;41(10):1769-75.

[59] Sader MA, Griffiths KA, McCredie RJ, et al. Androgenic anabolic steroids and arterial structure and function in male bodybuilders. *J Am Coll Cardiol.* 2001 Jan;37(1):224-30.

[60] Ebenbichler CF, Sturm W, Ganzer H et al. Flow mediated, endothelium-dependent vasodilatation is impaired in male body builders taking anabolic-androgenic steroids. *Atherosclerosis.* 2001 Oct;158(2):483-90.

[61] Miyachi M, Kawano H, Sugawara J, et al. Unfavorable effects of resistance training on central arterial compliance: a randomized intervention study. *Circulation.* 2004 Nov 2;110(18):2858-63.

[62] Rakobowchuk M, McGowan CL, de Groot PC, et al. Endothelial function of young healthy males following whole body resistance training. *J Appl Physiol.* 2005 Jun;98(6):2185-90.

[63] Kasikcioglu E, Oflaz H, Arslan A, et al. Aortic elastic properties in athletes using anabolic-androgenic steroids. *Int J Cardiol.* 2007 Jan 2;114(1):132-4.

[64] D'Ascenzo S, Millimaggi D, Di Massimo C, et al. Detrimental effects of anabolic steroids on human endothelial cells. *Toxicol Lett.* 2007 Mar 8;169(2):129-36.

[65] Ammar EM, Said SA, Hassan MS. Enhanced vasoconstriction and reduced vasorelaxation induced by testosterone and nandrolone in hypercholesterolemic rabbits. *Pharmacol Res.* 2004 Sep;50(3):253-9.

[66] McCrohon JA, Jessup W, Handelsman DJ, et al. Exposure increases human monocyte adhesion to vascular endothelium and endothelial cell expression of vascular cell adhesion molecule-1. *Circulation.* 1999;99(17):2317.

[67] Kaushik M, Sontineni S P & Hunter C. Cardiovascular disease and androgens: a review. *Int J Cardiol*, 2010142, 8-14.

[68] LeGros T, McConnell D, Murry T, et al.T he effects of 17 alpha-methyltestosterone on myocardial function in vitro. *Med Sci Sport Exerc.* 2000 May;32(5):897-903.

[69] Belhani D, Fanton L, Vaillant F, et al. Cardiac lesions induced by testosterone: protective effects of dexrazoxane and trimetazidine. *Cardiovasc Toxicol.* 2009 Jun;9(2):64-9.

[70] Boushey CJ, Beresford SA, Omenn GS & Motulsky AG. A quantitative assessment of plasma homocysteine as a risk factor for vascular disease. Probable benefits of increasing folic acid intakes. *JAMA.* 1995 Oct 4;274(13):1049-57.

[71] Zmuda JM, Bausserman LL, Maceroni D, Thompson PD. The effect of supraphysiologic doses of testosterone on fasting total homocysteine levels in normal men. *Atherosclerosis.* 1997 Apr;130(1-2):199-202.

[72] Ridker PM, Rifai N, Rose L, et al. Comparison of C-reactive protein and low-density lipoprotein cholesterol levels in the prediction of first cardiovascular events. *N Engl J Med.* 2002 Nov 14;347(20):1557-65.

[73] Grace FM, Davies B. Raised concentrations of C reactive protein in anabolic steroid using bodybuilders. *Br J Sports Med.* 2004 Feb;38(1):97-8.

[74] Arazi H, Ebrahmi M, Hosseini K. Effect of anabolic steroids consumption on c-reactive protein (CRP) in bodybuilders. *Payavard Salamat* 2011;4(2-4):43-49

[75] Barbosa J, Seal US, Doe RP. Effects of anabolic steroids on haptoglobin, orosmucoid, plasminogen, fibrinogen, transferrin, ceruloplasmin, alpha-1-antitrypsin, beta-glucuronidase and total serum proteins. *J Clin Endocrinol Metab,* 1971;33:388-398.

[76] Small M, McArdle BM, Lowe GD, et al. The effects of intramuscular stanozolol on fibrinolysis and blood lipids. *Thromb Res.* 1982;28:27-36.

[77] Verheijen JH, Rijken DC, Chang GT. Modulation of rapid plasminogen activator inhibitor in plasma by stanozolol. *Throm Haemost,* 1984;51:396-397.

[78] Shahidi NT. Androgens and erythropoiesis. *N Engl J Med,* 1973;289:72-80.

[79] Coviello AD, Kaplan B, Lakshman KM, et al.: Effects of graded doses of testosterone on erythropoiesis in healthy young and older men. *J Clin Endocrinol Metab* 93:914-9, 2008.

[80] Viallard JF, Marit G, Mercie P, et al. Polycythaemia as a complication of transdermal testosterone therapy. *Br J Haematol* 110:237-8, 2000.

[81] Dobs AS, Meikle AW, Arver S, et al. Pharmacokinetics, efficacy, and safety of a permeation-enhanced testerosterone in comparison with bi-weekly injections of testerosterone enanthate for the treatment of hypogonadal men. *J Clin Endocrinol Metab.* 1999;64:3469–78.

[82] Jockenhovel F, Vogel E, Reinhardt W, et al.: Effects of various modes of androgen substitution therapy on erythropoiesis. *Eur J Med Res* 2:293-8, 1997.

[83] Viallard JF, Marit G, Mercie P, et al. Polycythaemia as a complication of transdermal testosterone therapy. *Br J Haematol.* 2000;110:237–8.

[84] Kluft C, Preston FE, Malia RG, et al. Stanozolol-induced changes in fibrinolysis and coagulation in healthy adults. *Thromb Haemost* 1984;51:157-164

[85] Small M, McLean JA, McArdle BM, et al. Haemostatic effects of stanoxolol in elderly medical patients, *Thromb Res.* 1984:35:353-358

[86] Rosenlum WI, el-Sabban F, Nelson GH, et al. Effects in mice of testosterone and dihydrotestosterone on platelet aggregation in injured arterioles and ex vivo. *Thromb Res.* 1987 Mar 15;45(6):719-28.

[87] Winter JH, Fenech A, Bennett B. Prophylactic antithrombotic therapy with stanozolol in patients with familial antithrombin III deficiency. *Br J Haematol* 1984;57:527-537

[88] Ferenchick, G.S. (1991). AAS use and thrombosis- is there a connection? *Medical Hypotheses*, 35: 27-31.

[89] Ferenchick G, Schwartz D, Ball M, Schartz K (1992). Androgen-anabolic steroid abuse and platelet aggregation: a pilot study in weight lifters. *American Journal of Medical Science*, 303: 78-82.

[90] Ajayi AAL, Mathur R, Halushka PV. Testosterone increase human platelet thromboxane A2 receptor density and aggregation responses. *Circulation.* 1995;91:2742–7.

[91] Ansell JE, Tiarks C, Fairchild VK. Coagulation abnormalities associated with the use of anabolic steroids. *Am Heart J* 1993:125:367-371

[92] Ferenchick, G. S., Hirokawa, G., Mammen, E. F., Schwartz, K. A. (1995). Anabolic-androgenic steroid abuse in weight lifters: evidence for activation of the hemostatic system. *American Journal of Hematology*, 49: 282-288.

[93] Kahn NN, Sinha AK, Spungen AM, et al. Effects of oxandrolone, an anabolic steroid, on hemostasis. *Am J Hematol* 2006;81:95-100

[94] Stergiopoulos K, Brennan JJ , Mathews R, et al. Anabolic steroids, acute myocardial infarction and polycythemia: A case report and review of the literature. *J Vasc Health Risk Man* Nov 2008 4(6):1475-1480.

[95] Fried W, Gurney CW. The erythropoietic-stimulating effects of androgens. *Ann NY Acad Sci.* 1968;149:356–65.

[96] Winkler, U.H. (1996). Effects of androgens on haemostasis. *Maturitas*, 24: 147-155.

[97]	Frankle MA, Eichberg R, Zachariah SB. Anabolic androgenic steroids and a stroke in an athlete: case report. Arch Phys Med Rehabil. 1988 Aug;69(8):632-3.

[98]	Mochizuki RM, Richter KJ. Cardiomyopathy and Cerebrovascular Accident Associated with Anabolic-Androgenic Steroid Use. *Physician and Sportsmedicine*. 1988;16(11):109-11,14.

[99]	Kennedy MC, Corrigan AB, Pilbeam ST. Myocardial infarction and cerebral haemorrhage in a young body builder taking anabolic steroids. *Aust N Z J Med*. 1993 Dec;23(6):713.

[100] Akhter J, Hyder S, Ahmed M. Cerebrovascular accident associated with anabolic steroid use in a young man. *Neurology*. 1994 Dec;44(12):2405-6.

[101] Sahraian MA, Mottamedi M, Azimi AR, Moghimi B. Androgen-induced cerebral venous sinus thrombosis in a young body builder: case report. *BMC Neurol*. 2004 Dec 3;4(1):22.

[102] Santamarina RD, Besocke AG, Romano LM, Ioli PL, Gonorazky SE. Ischemic stroke related to anabolic abuse. *Clin Neuropharmacol*. 2008 Mar-Apr;31(2):80-5.

[103] Cooper I, Reeve N, Doherty W *BMJ Case Reports* Published 30 June 2011;published online 30 June 2011, doi:10.1136/bcr.02.2011.3857

[104] Shimada Y, Yoritaka A, Tanaka Y, et al. Cerebral Infarction in a Young Man Using High-dose Anabolic Steroids, *J Stroke Cardiovasc Dis*, Available online 8 September 2011

[105] Youssef MA, Alqallaf A, Abdella N *BMJ Case Reports* Published 4 July 2011;published online 4 July 2011, doi:10.1136/bcr.12.2010.3650

[106] Gaede JT, Montine TJ. Massive pulmonary embolus and anabolic steroid abuse. *JAMA*. 1992 May 6;267(17):2328-9.

[107] Alhadad A, Acosta S, Sarabi L, Kolbel T. Pulmonary embolism associated with protein C deficiency and abuse of anabolic-androgen steroids. *Clin Appl Thromb Hemost*.2010 Apr;16(2):228-31.

[108] Liljeqvist S, Hellden A, Bergman U, Soderberg M. Pulmonary embolism associated with the use of anabolic steroids. *Eur J Intern Med*. 2008 May;19(3):214-5.

[109] Laroche GP. Steroid anabolic drugs and arterial complications in an athlete—a case history. *Angiology*. 1990 Nov;41(11):964-9.

[110] Jaillard AS, Hommel M, Mallaret M. Venous sinus thrombosis associated with androgens in a healthy young man. *Stroke*. 1994 Jan;25(1):212-3.

[111] Mewis C, Spyridopoulos I, Kuhlkamp V, Seipel L. Manifestation of severe coronary heart disease after anabolic drug abuse. *Clin Cardiol.* 1996 Feb;19(2):153-5.

[112] Nieminen MS, Ramo MP, Viitasalo M, Heikkila P, Karjalainen J, Mantysaari M, et al. Serious cardiovascular side effects of large doses of anabolic steroids in weight lifters. *Eur Heart J.* 1996 Oct;17(10):1576-83.

[113] Palfi S, Ungurean A, Vecsei L. Basilar artery occlusion associated with anabolic steroid abuse in a 17-year-old bodybuilder. *Eur Neurol.* 1997;37(3):190-1.

[114] Falkenberg M, Karlsson J, Ortenwall P. Peripheral arterial thrombosis in two young men using anabolic steroids. *Eur J Vasc Endovasc Surg.* 1997 Feb;13(2):223-6.

[115] Hourigan LA, Rainbird AJ, Dooris M. Intracoronary stenting for acute myocardial infarction (AMI) in a 24-year-old man using anabolic androgenic steroids. *Aust N Z J Med.*1998 Dec;28(6):838-9.

[116] McCarthy K, Tang AT, Dalrymple-Hay MJ, Haw MP. Ventricular thrombosis and systemic embolism in bodybuilders: etiology and management. *Ann Thorac Surg.* 2000 Aug;70(2):658-60.

[117] Ment J, Ludman PF. Coronary thrombus in a 23 year old anabolic steroid user. *Heart.* 2002 Oct;88(4):342.

[118] Frogel JK, Weiss SJ, Kohl BA. Transesophageal echocardiography diagnosis of coronary sinus thrombosis. *Anesth Analg.* 2009 Feb;108(2):441-2.

[119] Urhausen A, Holpes R, Kindermann W. One- and two-dimensional echocardiography in bodybuilders using anabolic steroids. *Eur J Appl Physiol Occup Physiol.* 1989;58(6):633-40.

[120] Sachtleben TR, Berg KE, Elias BA, Cheatham JP, Felix GL, Hofschire PJ. The effects of anabolic steroids on myocardial structure and cardiovascular fitness. *Med Sci Sports Exerc.* 1993 Nov;25(11):1240-5.

[121] D'Andrea A, Caso P, Salerno G, et al. Left ventricular early myocardial dysfunction after chronic misuse of anabolic androgenic steroids: Doppler myocardial and strain imaging analysis. *Br J Sports Med.* 2007 Mar;41(3):149-55.

[122] Dickerman RD, Schaller F, McConathy WJ. Left ventricular wall thickening doesoccur in elite power athletes with or without anabolic steroid Use. *Cardiology.* 1998 Oct;90(2):145-8.

[123] Hartgens F, Cheriex EC, Kuipers H. Prospective echocardiographic assessment of androgenic-anabolic steroids effects on cardiac structure

and function in strength athletes. *Int J Sports Med.* 2003 Jul;24(5):344-51.

[124] Nottin S, Nguyen LD, Terbah M, Obert P. Cardiovascular effects of androgenic anabolic steroids in male bodybuilders determined by tissue Doppler imaging. *Am J Cardiol.*2006 Mar 15;97(6):912-5.

[125] Kasikcioglu E, Oflaz H, Umman B, Bugra Z. Androgenic anabolic steroids also impair right ventricular function. *Int J Cardiol.* 2009 May 1;134(1):123-5.

[126] Baggish AL, Weiner RB, Kanayama G, Hudson JI, Picard MH, Hutter AM, Jr., et al. Long-term anabolic-androgenic steroid use is associated with left ventricular dysfunction. *Circ Heart Fail.* 2010 Jul 1;3(4):472-6.

[127] Krieg A, Scharhag J, Kindermann W, Urhausen A. Cardiac tissue Doppler imaging in sports medicine. *Sports Medicine.* 2007;37(1):15-30.

[128] Lieberherr M, Grosse B. Androgens increase intracellular calcium concentration and inositol 1, 4, 5-trisphosphate and diacylglycerol formation via a pertussis toxin-sensitive G protein. *Journal of Biological Chemistry.* 1994;269(10):7217.

[129] Zaugg M, Jamali NZ, Lucchinetti E, Xu W, Alam M, Shafiq SA, et al. Anabolic androgenic steroids induce apoptotic cell death in adult rat ventricular myocytes. *Journal of Cellular Physiology.* 2001;187(1):90-5.

[130] Sullivan ML, Martinez CM, Gallagher EJ. Atrial fibrillation and anabolic steroids. *J Emerg Med.* 1999 Sep-Oct;17(5):851-7.

[131] Clark BM, Schofield RS. Dilated cardiomyopathy and acute liver injury associated with combined use of ephedra, gamma-hydroxybutyrate, and anabolic steroids. *Pharmacotherapy.* 2005 May;25(5):756-61.

[132] Stolt A, Karila T, Viitasalo M, Mantysaari M, Kujala UM, Karjalainen J. QT Interval and QT dispersion in endurance athletes and in power athletes using large doses of anabolic steroids. *Am J Cardiol.* 1999 Aug 1;84(3):364-6, A9.

[133] Bigi MA, Aslani A. Short QT interval: A novel predictor of androgen abuse in strength trained athletes. *Ann Noninvasive Electrocardiol.* 2009 Jan;14(1):35-9.

[134] Liu XK, Katchman A, Whitfield BH, Wan G, Janowski EM, Woosley RL, et al. Invivo androgen treatment shortens the QT interval and increases the densities of inward and delayed rectifier potassium currents in orchiectomized male rabbits. *Cardiovasc Res.* 2003 Jan;57(1):28-36.

[135] Sculthorpe N, Grace F, Jones P, Davies B. Evidence of altered cardiac electrophysiology following prolonged androgenic anabolic steroid use. *Cardiovasc Toxicol.* 2010 Dec;10(4):239-43.

[136] Bai, C. X.; Namekata, I.; Kurokawa, J.; Tanaka, H.; Shigenobu, K, & Furukawa, T. (2005). Role of nitric oxide in Ca2+ sensitivity of the slowly activating delayed rectifier K+current in cardiac myocytes. *Circ Res*, 96, 64-72.

[137] Bai, C. X.; Takahashi, K.; Masumiya, H.; Sawanobori, T.; & Furukawa, T. (2004). Nitric oxidedependent modulation of the delayed rectifier K+ current and the L-type Ca2+ current by ginsenoside Re, an ingredient of Panax ginseng, in guinea-pigcardiomyocytes. *Br J Pharmacol*, 142, 567-575.

[138] Fülöp L, Bányász T, Szabó G, Tóth IB, Bíró T, Lôrincz I, Balogh A, Petô K, Mikó I, Nánási PP 2006 Effects of sex hormones on ECG parameters and expression of cardiac ion channels in dogs. *Acta Physiol (Oxf)* 188:163-171.

[139] Maior AS, Menezes P, Pedrosa RC, Carvalho DP, Soares PP, Nascimento JH 2010 Abnormal cardiac repolarization in anabolic androgenic steroid users carrying out submaximal exercise testing. *Clin Exp Pharmacol Physiol* 37:1129-1133

[140] Medei E, Marocolo M, Rodrigues Dde C, Arantes PC, Takiya CM, Silva J, Rondinelli E, Goldenberg RC, de Carvalho AC, Nascimento JH 2010 Chronic treatment with anabolic steroids induces ventricular repolarization disturbances: cellular, ionic and molecular mechanism. *J Mol Cell Cardiol* 49:165-175

[141] Riezzo I, De Carlo D, Neri M, et al. Heart disease induced by AAS abuse, using experimental mice/rat models and the role of exercise-induced cardiotoxicity. *Mini Rev Med Chem.* 2011 May;11(5):409-24.

[142] Medei E, Marocolo M, de Carvalho Rodrigues D, et al. Chronic treatment with anabolic steroids induces ventricular repolarization disturbances: Cellular, ionic and molecular mechanism, *J Mol Cell Cardiol*, 2010;49(2):165-175

[143] Dodge T, Hoagland MF, The use of anabolic androgenic steroids and polypharmacy: a review of the literature, *Drug Alc Depend* 2011 114;(2-3):100-109.

[144] McNutt RA, Ferenchick GS, Kirlin PC, Hamlin NJ. Acute myocardial infarction in a 22-year-old world class weight lifter using anabolic steroids. *Am J Cardiol.* 1988 Jul 1;62(1):164.

[145] Bowman S. Anabolic steroids and infarction. *BMJ.* 1990 Mar 17;300(6726):750.

[146] Ferenchick GS, Adelman S. Myocardial infarction associated with anabolic steroid use in a previously healthy 37-year-old weight lifter. *Am Heart J.* 1992 Aug;124(2):507-8.

[147] Kennedy C. Myocardial infarction in association with misuse of anabolic steroids. *Ulster Med J.* 1993 Oct;62(2):174-6.

[148] Appleby M, Fisher M, Martin M. Myocardial infarction, hyperkalaemia and ventricular tachycardia in a young male body-builder. *Int J Cardiol.* 1994 Apr;44(2):171-4.

[149] Huie MJ. An acute myocardial infarction occurring in an anabolic steroid user. *Med Sci Sports Exerc.* 1994 Apr;26(4):408-13.

[150] Fisher M, Appleby M, Rittoo D, Cotter L. Myocardial infarction with extensive intracoronary thrombus induced by anabolic steroids. *Br J Clin Pract.* 1996 Jun;50(4):222-3.

[151] Goldstein DR, Dobbs T, Krull B, Plumb VJ. Clenbuterol and anabolic steroids: a previously unreported cause of myocardial infarction with normal coronary arteriograms. *South Med J.* 1998 Aug;91(8):780-4.

[152] Fineschi V, Baroldi G, Monciotti F, Paglicci Reattelli L, Turillazzi E. Anabolic steroid abuse and cardiac sudden death: a pathologic study. *Arch Pathol Lab Med.* 2001 Feb;125(2):253-5.

[153] Gunes Y, Erbas C, Okuyan E, Babalik E, Gurmen T. Myocardial infarction with intracoronary thrombus induced by anabolic steroids. *Anadolu Kardiyol Derg.* 2004 Dec;4(4):357-8.

[154] Angelilli A, Katz ES, Goldenberg RM. Cardiac arrest following anaesthetic induction in a world-class bodybuilder. *Acta Cardiol.* 2005 Aug;60(4):443-4.

[155] Wysoczanski M, Rachko M, Bergmann SR. Acute myocardial infarction in a young man using anabolic steroids. *Angiology.* 2008 Jun-Jul;59(3):376-8.

[156] Lunghetti S, Zaca V, Maffei S, Carrera A, Gaddi R, Diciolla F, et al. Cardiogenic shock complicating myocardial infarction in a doped athlete. *Acute Card Care.* 2009;11(4):250-1.

[157] Sullivan ML, Martinez CM, Gallagher EJ. Atrial fibrillation and anabolic steroids. *J Emerg Med.* 1999 Sep-Oct;17(5):851-7.

[158] Ahlgrim C, Guglin M. Anabolics and cardiomyopathy in a bodybuilder: case report and literature review. *J Card Fail.* 2009 Aug;15(6):496-500.

[159] Bispo M, Valente A, Maldonado R, Palma R, Gloria H, Nobrega J, et al. Anabolic steroid-induced cardiomyopathy underlying acute liver failure in a young bodybuilder. *World J Gastroenterol.* 2009 Jun 21;15(23):2920-2.

[160] Fineschi V, Riezzo I, Centini F, Silingardi E, Licata M, Beduschi G, et al. Sudden cardiac death during anabolic steroid abuse: morphologic and toxicologic findings in two fatal cases of bodybuilders. *Int J Legal Med.* 2007 Jan;121(1):48-53.

[161] Montischi M, Mazloum RE, Cecchetto G, et al. Anabolic androgenic steroid abuse and cardiac death in athletes: morphological and toxicological findings in four fatal cases. *Forensic Sci Internat,* Online 1 Nov 2011 ISSN 0379-0738

[162] Luke JL, Farb A, Virmani R, Sample RH. Sudden cardiac death during exercise in a weight lifter using anabolic androgenic steroids: pathological and toxicological findings. *J Forensic Sci.* 1990 Nov;35(6):1441-7.

[163] Campbell SE, Farb A, Weber KT. Pathologic remodeling of the myocardium in a weightlifter taking anabolic steroids. *Blood Press.* 1993 Sep;2(3):213-6.

[164] Hausmann R, Hammer S, Betz P. Performance enhancing drugs (doping agents) and sudden death--a case report and review of the literature. *Int J Legal Med.* 1998;111(5):261-4.

[165] Madea B, Grellner W. Long-term cardiovascular effects of anabolic steroids. *Lancet.* 1998 Jul 4;352(9121):33.

[166] Sivridis E, Pavlidis P, Stamos C, Giatromanolaki A, Sudden death after myocardial infarction in a high-school athlete. *J Forensic Sci* 2011 55;(5): 1378-1379

[167] Parssinen M, Kujala U, Vartiainen E, et al. Increased premature mortality of competitive powerlifters suspected to have used anabolic agents. *Int J Sports Med.* 2000;21:225–7.

In: Perspectives on Anabolic Androgenic ....   ISBN: 978-1-62081-243-3
Editors: F. Grace and J. S. Baker   © 2012 Nova Science Publishers, Inc.

Chapter 5

HEALTH AND BEHAVIOURAL CONSEQUENCES OF ANABOLIC ANDROGENIC STEROID (AAS) USE

Andrew McPherson[1,2], George Benson[2] and Colin R. Martin[,1]*

[1] chool of Health, Nursing and Midwifery,
University of the West of Scotland, UK
[2] Glasgow Addiction Service, Glasgow, UK

OVERVIEW OF CHAPTER

This chapter provides an analysis of anabolic-androgenic steroid (AAS) use and its impact on both the physical health and psychiatric consequences of the user. It begins with a brief introduction to the topic. This includes a definition and background for AAS. Different prevalence rates are highlighted and significant populations that use AAS are noted. A number of physical issues pertaining to AAS use are underscored and particular psychiatric consequences of AAS are analysed.

---

* Address for correspondence: Professor Colin R. Martin, School of Health, Nursing and Midwifery, University of the West of Scotland. Tel: 01292 886336; Fax: 01292 886327; E-mail: colin.martin@uws.ac.uk.

INTRODUCTION

Anabolic-androgenic steroids (AAS) is the broad term used to describe the male sex hormone testosterone and other endogenous androgenic hormones. It is also an expression used for synthesised products of these hormones [1]. The male sex hormone testosterone is primarily responsible for anabolic and androgenic effects highlighted in male childhood and adolescence [2]. AAS can be used legally, for example, prescribed as a treatment for delayed puberty and for conditions that may result in muscle wasting. There is however, significant concern at the non-prescribed use of these products and the use of these hormones in this context will be the primary focus of this chapter.

Synthetic products of testosterone occurred shortly after it was initially isolated in the 1930s [3]. Anabolic means simply to encourage tissue growth by increasing the metabolic process. Androgen is described as a group of steroid hormones that includes testosterone and dihydrotestosterone. The most abundant androgen is testosterone with 95% being secreted by the testicular Leydig cells. In addition to testosterone, the testes also secrete small amounts of the weak androgens droepiandrosterone and androstenedione [4].

The main source of these hormones is the testes. The hormones are responsible for male sexual features such as beard growth, deep voice and muscle development [5]. Anabolic steroids are synthetic forms of male hormones which include the drug nandrolone. Supraphysiologic doses of AAS combined with arduous exercise and good nutrition can cause users to unnaturally gain body muscle [6]. Nevertheless, the precise biological mechanisms responsible for these transformations remain unclear (Bahrke & Yesalis, 2004).

The lifetime prevalence of AAS use in the male population from the UK is reported to be 9.1% [7]. It is nevertheless reported that there is no accurate data on AAS use in the UK. It is believed though that most users fall into the 17 to 35 year-old age bracket and are usually male [8].

Meanwhile, in the US, male reported AAS use is said to be between 4% and 11% [9]. Other studies have shown a much lower prevalence rate of AAS use. For instance, Beaver and colleagues, in their research from a sample of young adult males from the US, showed only a 2.6% lifetime prevalence rate of AAS use and a 2.3% rate for use over the past year [10]. In Australian secondary school students, the lifetime prevalence rate was reported to be 2.4% of 12 to 17 year olds with use being more common in the 12 to 15 year old bracket [11]

A great deal of anecdotal evidence exists in the popular literature that point to AAS use among certain fraternities which are usually involved in sport and bodybuilding. This comes about from figures that highlight an historical prevalence rate of 75% for AAS use in homogeneous groups such as bodybuilders [12]. Research has tended to focus on professional athletes but attention is now being focused on other populations, such as male adolescents, with a particular emphasis on AAS use and aggression/violence [10]

Klotz and colleagues describe the use of AAS associated with a number of negative behaviours, such as; violence and criminality [13]. Prolonged AAS use can also have an impact on a number of psychological behaviours such as dependence issues and mood disorders [14]. AAS use may additionally increase or decrease libido in humans, have an impact on the cardiovascular system and can cause hepatic function changes to occur [2]. The behavioural consequences of AAS thus represent a complex psychobiology and therefore an appreciation of the physiological dimension to AAS is vital to understanding the behavioural aspects.

POTENTIAL HEALTH CONSEQUENCES OF AAS USE

The exact role of AAS use in the aetiology of a spectrum of diseases remains uncertain, although laboratory experiments have indicated an association with AAS use and risk factors for certain cancers, cardiovascular disease and infertility [2]. The potential physical health consequences of AAS use can be drawn from different systems of the body. Volkow (2006) [15] provides a detailed account of how AAS use can impact on the body's hormonal system, musculoskeletal system, cardiovascular system and the hepatic system. The author also states that AAS use may cause dermatological conditions and play a part in acquiring infections.

The manner in which AAS use may have consequences for the hormonal regulation can be split into gender categories. In males, it may cause infertility, breast development, shrinking of the testicles and male-pattern baldness. In females AAS may cause enlargement of the clitoris, unwanted body hair and may also cause male pattern baldness. If adolescents use AAS then the unnaturally elevated levels of testosterone and other sex hormones may provide indicators to prematurely stop growth. Another consequence of this is that it may cause tendons to rupture.

AAS use is associated with cardiovascular disease [2]. For instance, heart attacks and strokes have been known in individuals below the age of thirty who abuse steroids. Steroids can increase the level of low-density lipoprotein and decrease the level of high-density lipoprotein, which can increase the risk of atherosclerosis. Hepatic changes may also occur in individuals who abuse steroids. The most common hepatic feature of steroid abuse in the liver is hepatic carcinoma. AAS use may also cause an uncommon condition called peliosis hepatis; a vascular condition that affects the liver that causes blood-filled cavities in it. Cardiovascular risk factors in AAS use relate to a number of physiological changes including; raised concentrations of several clotting factors and alterations in the myocardium for example, increased left ventricular mass and dilated cardiomyopathy. Even though cardiovascular changes because of AAS use are serious, most effects can nevertheless be reversed on cessation of AAS [2].

Dermatological conditions such as severe acne and cysts can be caused by steroid abuse. Infections can occur in users who inject AAS. These infections can include viral infections such as; human immunodeficiency virus (HIV), hepatitis C (HCV) and hepatitis B (HBV). Other infections that steroid abusers acquire are endocarditis, and bacterial infections from injection sites. At some needle exchange schemes, AAS users account for a considerable amount of those who present there. This statistic is said to reflect the popularity of bodybuilding and the difficulty in obtaining suitable equipment for injecting oil-based steroids [8].

POTENTIAL PSYCHIATRIC CONSEQUENCES AF AAS USE

There remains a relative paucity of research on the emotional and behavioural impact of AAS use [16]. Chronic AAS use can nevertheless induce a number of psychiatric characteristics in users. The side-effects of AAS include; aggression, anxiety, depression, drug abuse and alter cognitive functioning. However adverse psychiatric effects of AAS such as confusion, paranoid delusion and hallucinations are said to be rare [8]. Chronic AAS use meanwhile is reported to interfere with the serotonergic and the dopaminergic systems [17]. Bahrke, & Yesalis (2004) [2] also underscore the psyche and behaviour changes as areas of concern in AAS users.

Serotonin (5-hydroxytryptamine) is described as a compound that acts like a neurotransmitter which has an essential influence on affect [5]. A reduction in serotonin is said to be linked with impulsivity rather than direct violence [18]. Dopamine also functions as a neurotransmitter. It can be used as a drug in heart failure, shock, severe trauma and septicaemia [5].

The behavioural effects of AAS use may be a consequence of secondary hormonal changes. The most common behavioural effect from AAS is irritability and aggression although it is hypothesised that not all anabolic steroids cause this. The numbers of extreme violence and behavioural disorders appear to be low but this may be due to underreporting or under-recognition of the issue. Even though AAS use may increase initial self-esteem or self-worth, severe mood-swings have been reported in some users which may eventually lead onto violence [19].

AGGRESSION AND VIOLENCE

It is suggested that the use of AAS is related to increased levels of violent behaviours [10]. This theory dates back to the mid-nineteenth century through the seminal work of Arnold Berthold. Berthold's experiments saw the aggression eliminated by the removal of testes from male chickens and subsequently reinstated when they were implanted with testes from donors [20]. The authors also report that there is a growing body of evidence available to suggest a clear link between anabolic steroid abuse and adverse psychological effects such as aggression. Nevertheless there remain inconsistencies in the literature and this may be due in part due to the illegal nature of the drugs. This may be consequential for reporting of illicit AAS use. In order to try and address the issue surrounding anabolic steroid abuse and aggression, researchers have developed animal modelling systems to try and create a controlled research environment.

The commonly abused AAS, nandrolone, has been shown to have an equivocal relationship with aggression and studies on rodents have shown the aggression outcome is variable, particularly in this population [20]. One hypothesis regarding this variation is that aggression may depend on experience or research environment. A system of taking anabolic androgens, known as stacking, may further compound problems. Stacking is where the AAS abuser takes more than one anabolic androgen at one time. This also usually means that individuals use AAS in a cyclical manner whereby they gradually titrate a dose of AAS before reducing it. Another name for the management of AAS in this way is called a pyramid [8].

One important point to consider is that although hormones may impact on aggressive behaviour, aggression can also impact on hormone concentrations. This reciprocal relationship is important for our understanding of the processes involved in AAS use. Moreover, there is an understanding that reactive aggression appears to be regulated by serotonin pathways while instrumental aggression is probably linked in some way to dopaminergic pathways [20]. The relationship that AAS use has with aggression is certainly complex [21]. It may be apparent in our understanding of this correlation that we tend to oversimplify it.

An essential component in steroid use and behaviour is reflected in adolescence. It has been recognised that AAS use by adolescents is increasing steadily and that adolescence is an important stage for learning and social behaviour development. It is documented that, "adolescence involves remodelling of steroid-sensitive neural circuits that mediate social behaviours" [22, p.328]. The authors conclude that AAS use is correlated with male sexual and agonistic behaviours and that this correlation is more pronounced if AAS use is initiated in adolescence.

Dependency: Only a small number of AAS users seek support and treatment for substance misuse. This may however increase in future years because those who initially used AAS are nearing middle age. This may bring many health concerns relating to AAS use into focus [23]. There is nevertheless debate surrounding the dependency issue of AAS. This deliberation focuses on the nosological criteria surrounding dependence and whether AAS use aligns itself to these conditions. Steroids do not appear to have an instant psychoactive effect, unlike other drugs of abuse and they do not appear to have traditional reinforcing characteristics of other drugs [8].

It is nevertheless argued that, AAS as a group of medicines have not been adequately researched. Interestingly, hypogonadism induced by AAS, appears to have similar criteria to an AAS dependency diagnosis [23]. It has also been hypothesised that AAS may have a similar psychological dependency category as other addictive drugs [9]. When users begin to take AAS, dependency appears to come about through the psychological process involved in muscle dysmorphia. As AAS use progresses, dependency resembles that of other drugs of addiction [24].

ANABOLIC-ANDROGENIC STEROID AND OTHER ILLICIT DRUG USE

AAS are on occasion used in conjunction with other illicit drugs. It is thought that AAS use can be a gateway to other illicit drugs but this hypothesis has not been confirmed. In their study of young people taken into custody for violent behaviour in Sweden, Gårevik & Rane (2010) [25] found that opiods were rarely used along with AAS. Cocaine was the preferred drug of choice in this group. This finding is not comparable with others studies. Kanayama and colleagues hypothesise that AAS use often leads to opiod and other psychotropic drug use [26]. Cocaine use has also been the subject of research. This examination has looked into the cardiotoxic effects of the two drugs used simultaneously [27]. Moreover, long-term, high-dose AAS use may lead to the use of other drugs [28]. There is a strong correlation between AAS users and other illicit drugs, such as heroin or other opiods. This may come about because a number of AAS users have reported using opiods to neutralise the effects of the AAS like irritability and insomnia [15]. Cannabis has also been shown to have a particular relationship with AAS but this may be due to cannabis being the most widely available illicit drug [25]. In a review of AAS use and other drugs, it concludes that individuals who experiment with AAS are more likely to experiment alcohol and other illicit drugs, although interestingly the authors find the relationship between AAS use and cannabis unclear [29].

BODY DYSMORPHIA

Muscle dysmorphia is a type of body dysmorphic disorder in which there is a pathological preoccupation with masculinity. Body dysmorphic disorder is defined as, "a preoccupation with an imagined defect in one's appearance. Alternatively, if a slight physical anomaly is present, the person's concern is markedly excessive" [30 p.267]. Muscle dysmorphia has been correlated strongly in weight lifters who abuse AAS [31]. Body dysmorphia in weight lifters has also been dubbed 'reverse anorexia' described as a fear of having a small and weak physique [32]. A strong physique and desirable body image has been linked to an increase in self-esteem and self-confidence, although many psychological affects may be potentially damaging to the individual [33] Muscle dysmorphia has also been linked with initial AAS dependency, although latterly AAS dependence displays classic signs of drug dependence [34].

Positive experiences of AAS might be an increase in self-confidence along with an improvement in strength and energy. Nevertheless, a degree of paranoia and psychosis have been highlighted in individuals who abuse AAS [2]. An affective state has been reported in some AAS users who stop using them. This has been linked to a state similar to withdrawal from alcohol or opiods (Kashkin, & Kleber, 1989). Those with perceived high self-esteem were less likely to engage in AAs use than those with perceived low self-esteem. Low self-esteem in adolescents was also believed to be of greater importance in AAS use than gender or race [35].

CONCLUSION

As we have seen a number of different populations are related to AAS use. These include adolescents, bodybuilders, weight lifters and professional athletes. Lifetime AAS prevalence rates can be confusing and this may be due in part to the prohibited nature of AAS. AAS use brings with it a number of health concerns that relate to systems of the body. Cardiovascular disease is particularly pertinent as is side-effects that result from male sex hormones such as breast development and infertility. Psychiatric effects of AAS use are also significant. Its use has been linked to aggression, although this relationship is complex and probably includes environmental factors and genetic influences. Significant psychiatric effects also include a unique form of body dysmorphia called muscle dysmorphia. AAS is also used as a gateway into other illicit drug use and in particular cocaine use. It is worth noting that we may see more unwanted effects of AAS use in the next few years as initial users become middle-aged.

REFERENCES

[1]   Marshall, E. (1998). The drug of champions. *Science, 242*(4876), 183-184.

[2]   Bahrke, M.S., & Yesalis, C.E. (2004). Abuse of anabolic androgenic steroids and related substances in sport and exercise. *Current Opinion in Psychopharmacology, 4*(6), 614-620.

[3]   David, K., Dingemanse, E., Freud, J., & Laquer, E. (1935). Uber Krystallinisches Hormon Hoden (Testosteron), wirksamer als aus Harn oder Cholesterin Bereitetes Androsteron. *Zeit. Physiol. Chem, 233*, 281-282.

[4]   Braunstein, G.D. (2001). Testes. In F.S. Greenspan & D.G. Gardner (Eds.), basic and Clinical Endocrinology (pp. 422-452). New York: Lange Medical Books/McGraw-Hill.

[5]   Martin, E.A. (2007). *Oxford Concise Colour Medical Dictionary* (3rd ed.). Oxford: Oxford University Press.

[6]   Kouri, E.M., Pope, H.G., Katz, D.L., & Oliva, P. (1995). Fat-free mass index in users and nonusers of anabolic-androgenic steroids. *Clinical Journal of Sport Medicine, 5*, 223-228.

[7]   Korkia, P., & Stimpson, G.V. (1997). Indications of prevalence, practice and effects of anabolic steroid use in Great Britain. *International Journal of Sports Medicine, 18*, 557-562.

[8]   Ghodse, H. (2002). *Drugs and Addictive Behaviour: A Guide to Treatment.* Cambridge: Cambridge University Press.

[9]   Brower, K.J. (1992). Clinical assessment and treatment of anabolic steroid users. *Psychiatric Annals, 22*, 35-40.

[10] Beaver, K.M., Vaughn, M.G., DeLisi, M., & Wright, J.P. (2008). Anabolic-Androgenic Steroid Use and Involvement in Violent Behavior in a Nationally Representative Sample of Young Adult Males in the United States. *American Journal of Public Health, 98*(12), 2185-2187.

[11] Dunn, M., & White, V. (2011). The epidemiology of anabolic-androgenic steroid use among Australian secondary school students. *Journal of Science and Medicine in Sport, 14*, 10-14.

[12] Lindström, M., Nilsson, A.L., Katzman, P.L., Janzon, L., & Dymling, J.-F. (1990). Use of anabolic-androgenic steroids among body builders – frequency and attitudes. *Journal of Internal Medicine, 227*(6), 407-411.

[13] Klotz, F., Petersson A., Hoffman, O., & Thiblin, I. (2010). The significance of anabolic androgenic steroids in a Swedish prison population. *Comprehensive Psychiatry, 51*, 312-318.

[14] Kanayama, G., Hudon J.I., & Pope H.G. (2008). Long-Term Psychiatric and Medical Consequences of Anabolic-Androgenic Steroid Abuse: A Looming Public Health Concern? *Drug and Alcohol Dependence, 98*(1-2), 1-12. doi: 10.1016/j.drugalcdep.2008.05.004.

[15] Volkow, N.D. (2006). Anabolic Steroid Abuse. *National Institute on Drug Abuse.* Retrieved from *http://www.nida.nih.gov/PDF/RRSteroids. pdf*

[16] Trenton, A.J., & Currier, G.W. (2005). Behavioral manifestations of anabolic steroid use. *CNS Drugs, 18*, 571-595.

[17] Elfverson, M., Johansson, T., Zhou, Q., Le Grevès, P., & Nyberg, F. (2011). Chronic administration of the anabolic steroid nandrolone alters neurosteroid action at the sigma-1 receptor but not at the sigma-2 or NMDA receptors. Neuropharmacology, doi: 10.1016/j.neuropharm. 2011.01.005.

[18] Gelder, M.G., Andreasen, N.C., Lopez-Ibor, J.J., & Geddes, J.R. (2000) *New Oxford Textbook of Psychiatry*. Oxford: Oxford University Press.

[19] Pope, H.G., & Katz, D.L. (1988). Affective and psychotic symptoms associated with anabolic steroid use. *American Journal of Psychiatry, 145*(5), 487-490.

[20] Trainor, B.C., Sisk, C.L., & Nelson, R.J. (2009). Hormones and the Development and Expression of Aggressive Behavior. In D.W. Pfaff, A.P. Arnold, A.M. Etgen, S.E. Fahrbach & R.T. Rubin (Eds.), *Hormones, Brain and Behavior* (pp.167-203). San Diego: Academic Press.

[21] Beel, A., maycock, B., & McLean, N. (1988). Current perspective on anabolic steroids. *Drug and Alcohol Review, 17*, 87-103.

[22] Salas-Ramirez, K.Y., Montalto, P.R., & Sisk, C.L. (2009). Anabolic steroids have long-lasting effects on male social behaviors. *Behavioural Brain Research, 208*, 328-335.

[23] Scally, M.C., & Tan, R.S. (2009). Complexities in Clarifying the Diagnostic Criteria for Anabolic-Androgenic Steroid Dependence. *American Journal of Psychiatry, 166*(10), 1187.

[24] Kanayama, G., Brower, K.J., Wood, R.I., Hudson, J.I., & Pope H.G. (2009). Issues for DSM-V: Clarifying the diagnostic criteria for anabolic-androgenic steroid dependence. *American Journal of Psychiatry, 166*(6), 642-644.

[25] Gårevik, N., & Rane, A. (2010). Dual use of anabolic-androgenic steroids and narcotics in Sweden. *Drug and Alcohol Dependence, 109*, 144-146.

[26] Kanayama, G., Cohane, G.H., Weiss, R.D., Pope, H.G. (2003) Past anabolic-androgenic steroid use among men admitted for substance abuse treatment: an under recognized problem? *Journal of Clinical Psychiatry, 64*, 156-160.

[27] Melchert, R.B. & Welder, A.A. (1992). Cardiotoxic effects of cocaine and anabolic-androgenic steroids in the athlete. *Journal of Pharmacological and Toxicological Methods, 29*(2), 61-68.

[28] Kashkin, K.B., & Kleber, H.D. (1989). Hooked on hormones? An anabolic steroid addiction hypothesis. *Journal of the American Medical Association, 262*, 3166-3170.

[29] Dodge, T., & Hoagland, M.F. (2011). The use of anabolic androgenic steroids and polypharmacy: A review of the literature. *Drug and Alcohol Dependence, 114*, 100-109.

[30] Veale, D. (2002). Shame in body dysmorphic disorder. In P. Gilbert & J. Miles (Eds.), *Body Shame: Conceptualisation, Research and Treatment* (pp. 267-282). Hove: Brunner-Routledge.

[31] Olivardia, R., Pope, H.G., & Hudson, J.I. (2000) Muscle dysmorphia in male weightlifters: A case-control study. *The American Journal of Psychiatry*, 157(8), 1291-1296.

[32] Pope, H.G., Katz, D.L., & Hudson, J.I. (1993). Anorexia nervosa and "reverse anorexia" among 108 male bodybuilders. *Comprehensive Psychiatry*, *34*, 406-409.

[33] Wroblewska, A-M. (1996). Androgenic-anabolic steroids and body dysmorphia in young men. *Journal of Psychosomatic Research*, *42*(3), 225-234.

[34] Kanayama, G., Brower, K.J., Wood, R.I., Hudson, J.I., & Pope H.G. (2010). Treatment of anabolic-androgenic steroid dependence: Emerging evidence and its implications. *Drug and Alcohol Dependence*, *109*, 6-13.Denham, B.E. (2010).

[35] Adolescent self-perceptions and attitudes toward school as determinants of anabolic-androgenic steroid risk estimates and normative judgements. *Youth & Society*, doi: 10.1177/0044118x10379736.

In: Perspectives on Anabolic Androgenic ....   ISBN: 978-1-62081-243-3
Editors: F. Grace and J. S. Baker   © 2012 Nova Science Publishers, Inc.

Chapter 6

WHATEVER HAPPENED TO EVERYONE TRAINING HARD, PLAYING HARD AND WHOEVER WAS THE BEST WON FAIR AND SQUARE? (SOCIOLOGICAL VOICES ON THE USE OF BANNED SUBSTANCES)

Alex McInch, Scott Fleming and Anna Leyshon
Cardiff Metropolitan University, Cardiff, UK

ABSTRACT

This chapter presents a sociological investigation into the perceptions of, and opinions about those involved in elite level sports concerning the use performance enhancing drugs. An interpretivist approach was adopted that sought to highlight the real life experiences of key stake-holders from the elite level of one particular high-profile, multi-event sport. The 'sociological voices' were crafted into non-fictional narratives and include contributions from an international competitor inexperienced at senior level, three Olympians, a Paralympian, an elite level specialist coach, and a senior administrator – of these, two were female. The data are presented in this way to synthesise the findings into an accessible form, and protect the anonymity of those involved. The main themes to emerge from the interviews and presented in the narratives include: the pressures and responsibilities of being an elite performer, the relation of performance to financial security, the fairness and integrity of sports, the perception of variable robustness of testing amongst different countries, differences between junior level and senior competition and between men and women.

Keywords: Performance enhancing drugs; non-fictional narratives; sociological voices

INTRODUCTION

The issues and questions associated with the use of banned performance enhancing substances in elite level sports are never far away. A quick Internet search for "drugs in sports" reveals a number of prominent recent controversies from a variety of sports. In early 2011, there was a positive test in the Tour de France [1][1], and a three-year ban for a British male shot-putter who had also coached at the 2008 Paralympics [2]. Whether or not the involvement of the individuals concerned is a matter of particular surprise within their respective sporting communities is arguable; but the revelations that these sports are once again in the spotlight will hardly send shock waves through the world of sport more generally.

Other sports less commonly associated with the use of banned performance enhancing substances have also recently received the sort of attention that inevitably tarnishes their image. Sri Lankan cricketer Upul Tharanga tested positive and was banned by the International Cricket Council [3], five players from Mexico's men's football squad were suspended from the Concacaf Gold Cup in the USA [4], and two UK-based rugby union players were banned by a Rugby Football Union disciplinary panel [5]. What is clear, therefore, is that the use of banned substances by human participants is practised in a number of different sports[2].

Even the more responsible "broadsheet" reporting of "drugs in sports" at the high-quality end of the print media in Britain can begin to resemble "moral

---

[1] This is separate from the other controversies about two of the sport's biggest names, Lance Armstrong and Alberto Contador, which (at the time of writing – July 2011) look set to last for some considerable time and further damage the reputation of professional cycling and the iconic Tour de France event.

[2] There is a separate discussion altogether about the use of banned substances in sports involving animals. It has been alleged in one account reported in The Guardian newspaper that the British horse racing industry includes "plenty of trainers" using banned substances on their horses [30].

panic", and those found guilty demonised into "folk devils" [6]. The broadcast media are similar but the immediacy of the coverage can often sensationalise the news item further still.

More scholarly and conceptually sophisticated accounts of the use of banned substances include historical contextualisation [7;8], scientific analysis [9], policy evaluation and critique [10], as well as considerations of the ethical dimensions of the practices of "doping" [11], all of which contribute to an understanding of their impact on the global domain of sport. Importantly, though, whilst many scholars, commentators and journalists have offered opinion on drugs in sport, consideration of the competing arguments from within sport has received relatively little attention. In this chapter, we seek to address this by providing a series of sociological voices to illuminate the debates. We do so by creating some non-fictional narratives based on a series of in-depth interviews with key actors in a high profile, multi-event Olympic and Paralympic sport.

In part the narratives speak for themselves, but like Stewart *et al.* (2010) [12], we are keen to avoid misunderstanding and misinterpretation in the reading of the narratives. Hence we provide a (necessarily brief) analysis of the key themes and issues after each one. We begin with an account of the research design, and conclude the chapter with a short summary.

RESEARCH DESIGN

The research presented in this chapter is in a style of doing and reporting empirical findings that has received increasing interest during the last decade. Underpinned by an epistemological commitment to interpretivism, it emerged in part as a reaction to the hegemonic dominance of positivism [13] and allows for the potential emergence of socially constructed multiple "truths" [14]. Qualitative researchers adopt a wider (and growing) range of styles of representation that challenge conventional modes of formal "scientific" writing [15,16]. For instance, there are confessional tales, autoethnographies, poetic representations, ethnodramas. Some of these have inevitably generated questions about their legitimacy and the evaluation of their quality [17] – and not just amongst those who are hostile to their epistemological foundations.

For this study, however, our preferred approach was the use of non-fictional narratives in the form of storytelling. This had the multiple virtues of: (i) being grounded in well-established research protocols that generate data [18]; (ii) being based on a set of authentic experiences, views and opinions of the "actors" involved [19]; (iii) maintaining the anonymity of those involved and of the sport when dealing with some well-known personalities[3] and a topic of considerable sensitivity [20]; (iv) making accessible to a wide-ranging set of audiences material that might be more impenetrable if depicted using other (more conventional and traditional) modes of representation[4].

A "thumbnail sketch" of two studies that adopted a similar approach help to illustrate. First, Carless and Sparkes (2008) [18] investigated the physical activity experiences of men with a serious mental illness. They presented three short creative non-fiction vignettes that best represented these experiences. The severity of the condition at times led to fragmentary and disjointed responses by the participants, and the authors adopted Agar's (1995) [21] notion of "authorial presence" to formulate a coherent and smooth text that preserved the original context of the remarks. Second, in a study of gender relations and notions of femininity in trampoline gymnastics, Stewart et al. (2010) [12] presented two narrative tales that highlighted perceptions of surveillance and self-regulation for the young female participants. The explicit commitment to an anonymised non-fictional narrative provided an opportunity to express opinions away from the sport's institutional gaze. In both cases well-established methods of data collection enabled the narratives to be constructed. Faithful to the contexts and the authenticity of the participants' accounts, these studies made accessible the (relatively) inaccessible [18] and created the opportunity for the uninhibited expression of opinions [12].

These principles shaped the design of the present study. Through a combination of sampling techniques (opportunity, purposive and snow-ball), initial contact was made with a total of five participants. These included an international competitor inexperienced at senior level, three Olympians, a Paralympian, an elite level specialist coach, and a senior administrator. Of these, two were female.

---

[3] The problem of disclosure in some forms of qualitative research has been addressed elsewhere. For instance, Mellick and Fleming (2010) [31] have noted that Tsang's (2000) [32] account of her career as an Olympic rower cannot conceal the other persons involved (they are a matter of public record) without the power of the narrative being lost. However through skilful story-telling the other key actors are identifiable individually and their anonymity is assured.

[4] It is our view that one of the major advantages of the 'alternative' modes of presentation currently finding favour with qualitative researchers in sport studies is precisely this – to make accessible to interested audiences (and perhaps the less interested too) material that might otherwise be consigned to the scholarly journal. That is to say, too often academics use mainly the established conventions and esoteric vocabulary of an academic discipline to communicate with fellow academics from within the same discipline. Inevitably other potential 'end-users' of the research are either neglected or excluded.

Informed consent was granted and each participant was interviewed for between one and two hours. The interviews were recorded digitally and a content analysis of the raw data was conducted. Finally, adopting Maykut and Moorhouse's (1994) [22] guidance, the data were analysed to ensure that meaning was conveyed under the initial formation of the original themes. Three creative non-fictional texts were then produced to represent the data, and the participants were invited to comment on them and to indicate their contentment with the inclusion of the narratives in this chapter – all did so without comment except to support the interpretation and depiction of their experiences as they had described them.

Scenario 1: "Us girls don't talk about it that much"

Twenty year old Anya arrived at her first senior international training camp. The multipurpose sports venue and surrounding facilities were awesome, she'd never seen anything like it. There was a 50m swimming pool, access to the river, multi-use sports hall, a state-of-the-art weights room and separate cardio gym, a red bouncy tartan track, brand new astroturf and endless fields. Between her gruelling workouts Anya spent time talking and drinking coffee with her senior team mate, Sarah. Anya had already learnt a lot from Sarah and their chats had become an important part of Anya's "apprenticeship" into elite level sport. As they sipped their coffee overlooking the waterfront on a warm sunny morning, Sarah was keen to find out how Anya was coping with the "step-up" from age-group training and competition. "So how are you finding it with the seniors?"

"It's fantastic. I'm learning so much", Anya replied enthusiastically. "...To be more sensible and to stay healthy and injury free by listening to my body. I guess I know about myself better and also about all the expectations that come with the sport... I was listening to the guys talking about drugs this morning and all the testing. It was really interesting – and new to me. Do you get tested much, Sarah?"

Sarah knew they'd have this conversation sooner or later. "Yes" she replied, "I'm tested regularly, I'm happy to be tested because I'm clean. But sometimes I do get annoyed when I have to get up at six in the morning. My other half is also involved in the sport and we've discussed it. We get frustrated, it's intrusive. But we're ok with it because we're clean." Sarah knew she sounded indignant, but made no apology.

Anya had never been tested and was a bit taken aback – "I've never been through it, how scary …" she mused. Sarah sensed Anya's unease and tried to reassure her: "Yeah, I suppose it is not very dignified. But one of the main things as a senior is to organise your location and let the testers know where you are. You have to control the environment."

"I know", Anya confirmed. Sarah had been involved in this kind of conversation before, she continued, "It is all very well in Britain because we're tested all the time, but if the rest of the world aren't doing it, it's not going to change anything. That's when it's not really fair.

"Aren't the other countries as strict?" Anya asked sensing her own naïveté. Without pausing to let Sarah answer she carried on, "I suppose it is always in the back of your mind that people from other countries might be taking drugs then. It's not something I'd consider. You're cheating yourself and the whole system. It's not fair on those who put in the hard work."

Sarah agreed and tried to make sense of the situation, "I think for anyone who gets to that stage, it's more than winning. It's about winning and getting sponsorship and fame and money. It seems to me that if you get to that point you're probably not thinking rationally. I think it's probably a kind of last resort. It's desperation. There's always an excuse for taking it, but that's all it is – an excuse. They say they're one step ahead of testers, but I think they're bound to get caught in the end."

Anya seemed to understand, "They'll have to pay the price in the end." "Absolutely," Sarah concurred. "And you don't know the long-term impact of taking drugs after their ban is over – that's why I think they should be banned for life." "And the temptation of doing it again", Anya added.

Confident that she'd got her message across, Sarah paused and reflected on the issue more generally. "You know Anya, what's really interesting is that we're sat here having this conversation, but the girls don't really talk about drugs that much … And it's not something I ever really come across. I mean I wouldn't even have a clue where to get it from. Us girls don't talk about it that much."

She remembered vividly another training camp, "Once, when we were in a camp with another country, there was a row of vitamins – at least I think they were vitamins. I didn't know what they were and didn't know whether they were banned substances or not. But they were all taking them – the boys and the girls."

At this point other squad members approached Anya and Sarah. Before they arrived Sarah took the opportunity to share some 'sisterly' advice, "You're a star of the future. Remember to manage the responsibilities that come with being a star. And remember that there's a life after sport. Never get to the stage where you'd do anything – even die for your sport. It's not worth it."

Anya was a neophyte member of the senior squad and her innocence was both surprising and endearing. Career progress from the junior ranks marked some major changes for her, and she was clearly awe-struck by the environment in which she found herself. Sarah acted in an informal mentor role to Anya and their conversations were part of a process of Anya's socialisation into the ethos and culture of the sport [23].

The use of banned substances did not feature in the day-to-day discourses of the female competitors, and together, Anya and Sarah shared an embodied commitment[5] to "fair play" [24]. For though Sarah acknowledged that the British testing procedures were inconvenient, it was important to her that Anya understood their importance for protecting the integrity of their sport. Inevitably Sarah had concerns that in countries where she thought the out-of-competition testing were less rigorous than in Britain, there was a possibility that the apparently successful competitors were actually drugs cheats.

Scenario 2: 'People's livelihoods are at stake'

It was a beautiful, hot spring morning in the Spanish sun on the first day of a national squad training camp. In the breakfast hall of a huge, multi-purpose sports complex there was an air of expectation – for many it could have been a pivotal year of elite competition. The plentiful buffet had the usual selections of fresh fruit, cereal and fruit juice, which were accompanied by a vast array of hot food selections. There was something for every appetite and dietary requirement. Nick, one of the well-established coaches, strolled in first and was followed shortly afterwards by Brian, one of his 'flock', as he liked to call them. They both chose their food and shuffled over to one of the empty tables in the middle of the room. They sat down, faced each other and started to eat.

"So, how are you feeling? Good sleep?" Nick asked Brian, who pondered for a few seconds before answering.

"Yeah not bad, just can't wait to get stuck into this training camp now".

Nick nodded in polite agreement but noticed that Brian appeared uneasy.

---

[5] See, for example, the interesting and well argued analyses of embodiment in sport [33;34]

"Are you sure everything's ok pal?" He enquired, and then continued light-heartedly in the mock tone of fatherly interest, "Come on, what's the matter?" Despite the humour there was a serious edge to Nick's genuine concern. An awkward silence followed. It lasted only seconds but seemed much longer. Eventually Brian replied hesitantly:

"I'm just...well...really pissed off, I feel like I want to punch someone."

Nick paused, he wasn't expecting that. "Well, tell me, what's the problem?" It was an open invitation for Brian to lay all his cards on the table. Nick was more than a coach to Brian, they had become friends and Nick was a listener and confidant for Brian.

"The thing is," Brian explained, "I've been hearing things about certain people that they have been on the gear, and to be honest it disgusts me. Why should I put every ounce of effort into my training and preparation and want to give a good account of myself staying clean when some idiot gets away with it and walks away with all the glory...? You know, I have a family to feed and bills to pay just like we all do, I don't think people realise sometimes that it's not just about winning and losing, it's much more complex than that, people's livelihoods are at stake".

Nick listened attentively, taking a few moments to digest what Brian has just told him. This scenario was all too familiar for Nick and he thought he had an answer to ease Brian's anger:

"Well, believe it or not I know exactly how you feel. When I was competing back in the early 90s, it was rife, and I openly knew that certain competitors were taking performance enhancers, it even got to the stage where there were tablets floating around liberally, I even had some in my hand one day. But I thought no, why should I ruin all of my hard work with one silly mistake? I feel proud that I came into the sport far later than others, I was clean and still got to where I did. I know that I could make a phone call right now and arrange for you to take certain things that would almost certainly improve certain areas of your training, but I know your frustration doesn't lie with you taking gear. It's with the ones that do and get away with it, but unfortunately that's part of the sport. People know how to beat the system and if they feel that they can get away with it, they'll try it".

Brian was stunned with this revelation. He knew that Nick had competed at the very highest level and had always respected him for that. But he never knew exactly what Nick thought, and why he thought it. He didn't realise that Nick had been challenged by exactly the same frustrations that he was experiencing. Brian was surprisingly relieved and reassured. He sat back in his chair and was satisfied with what Nick had shared with him.

Another silent moment passed. "Come on, we've got a long day ahead of us" Nick cajoled as he slapped Brian on the back warmly. They put their trays on the trolley and left the dining hall for training. Brian felt content.

As an experienced male competitor Brian was angry and frustrated about the rumours that some fellow competitors were using banned substances. His was a sense of injustice because of the very real human consequences that transcended the sport itself, and affected others as well as himself.

The financial imperatives of properly supporting his family weighed heavily upon him [25], and he was constantly aware the precarious nature of his source of income.

Nick's own attitude to banned substances had been shaped by his own history and biography in the sport [26]. His was an uncomplicated argument about the consequences of getting caught – and like other coaches he knew, he would have had no difficulty in getting access to banned performance enhancers had he wanted to.

Nick was a pragmatist and, on the face of it displayed an unsophisticated level of moral reasoning [27]. Yet he was also proud of having been a 'clean' competitor and having achieved his own success within the rules and spirit of sport.

Scenario 3: 'What happened to our sporting virtues?'

A meeting for a small group of senior sport administrators had just drawn to a close in the conference suite of a large city-centre hotel. The proposed agenda for the meeting had been linked to the strategic direction of the sport, but a more pressing matter had emerged in recent days with breaking news of another doping scandal – a senior squad member, Dale, had tested positive for a banned anabolic-androgenic steroid. It had become crucial to limit the reputational damage to the sport and the importance of the meeting was magnified because a major international multi-sport event was only months away. Lionel, one of the most senior figures in the sport, made his way to the hotel lounge with Derek, another key figure in the organisation. As they sat down and ordered coffee they looked relieved to be able to relax. It had been a mentally draining first half to the meeting. Both had been elite level competitors some years ago and had been team-mates. Derek made eye contact with Lionel and broke the silence:

"How was that for you? ... I have to say that that silly git [Dale, who had tested positive] has tarnished us all again. When's this going to stop? It wasn't even on the radar in our day, whatever happened to everyone training hard, playing hard and whoever was the best won fair and square? What happened to our sporting virtues?"

"Yes", Lionel added. "The trouble is, with all of the financial incentives in the sport it's no wonder that some of them are going to try and gain that advantage over an opponent, especially if they're not going to get caught for something they shouldn't be doing. They're fast becoming hot commodities and they've got a lot at stake for the short time they're at the elite level." Derek nodded in partial agreement, but offered another thread to the discussion.

"That's true, but it's down to our governing body that Dale was caught..." Lionel interrupted respectfully:

"Wait a minute Derek, Dale was reported by someone not even linked to the governing body. If that never happened then he probably wouldn't have got caught and we would have been none the wiser. Sometimes I feel that the sport is just a breeding ground for cheating because of all the money and fame on offer".

Paradoxically, the conversation they were now having was exactly the kind of discussion that had been needed in the meeting that had just adjourned. Derek knew Lionel's perspective well – this wasn't the first time they'd had a conversation like this, but he was still keen to make his own particular point:

"But I still think that a ban for life is the only way forward in these situations, I think they're starting to realise the full impact of the wrong-doing. After all, we have a duty of care in the messages we send out to youngsters involved at grassroots level, they have to realise that this is wrong, completely unacceptable and has no place in sport". Lionel nodded in agreement, but questioned Derek's viewpoint on punishment:

"I think we're slowly winning the battle, but we have to contextualise things here. A drink-driver can get caught, potentially cause lots of physical, emotional and structural damage, be punished, banned for a year or so and be back driving again. I think that's far worse in the grand scheme of things. We need to realign with the fact that in this country, you do the crime and you do the time".

The attitude of neither man surprised the other. They sipped their coffee and gave each other a grin of approval. Moments later they'd finished and walked to the conference suite to reconvene for the second half of the meeting for what promised to be a contentious couple of hours.

Derek and Lionel were former participants, as sports administrators often are. As key figures in the sport, their influence on the organisational culture was significant and disproportionate [28]. They brought to their respective roles their experiences as elite level competitors, but not in the present era of commercialised professional sport.

Yet they recognised the temptations for elite competitors – for the winners in high-profile global competitions, there was fame and financial security for life.

Whilst committed to what they saw as the proper spirit of sport, they were also concerned about the reputational damage that bad publicity brought to the sport. Derek had a straightforward approach to dealing with competitors who got caught using banned substances – a ban for life. Lionel's was a more nuanced understanding, sensitive to context, and reflected a wider perspective of sport in society more generally [29][6].

CONCLUSION

This chapter attempted to illuminate some of the arguments about the use of banned substances in sport by drawing upon some empirical research with key stake-holders in a high-profile multi-event sport. The views expressed are not an exhaustive account of all competitors, coaches and administrators in that sport; rather, they are indicative of those held by some. We do not claim that these views are representative in any way, but neither do we have any reason to think that they are not shared by others. Ours is not, therefore, an argument for generalisability.

The usage of non-fictional narratives to represent the participants' voices was a deliberate attempt to make the work accessible to a wider set of audiences than is often the case in academic circles – though we recognise that a book of this kind is unlikely to be the most effective mechanism to secure that outcome in any case. Importantly though, the narratives require some interpretation. As Stewart *et al.* (2010) [12] explain, when the subject matter is sensitive (as work on banned substances in sport undoubtedly is), it is important to avoid ambiguity and misunderstanding. Hence, the short commentaries that follow each of the narratives make explicit the key themes[7].

In summary, from this study it seems that:

1. The spirit of sport (based on 'fair play' and natural justice) remains potent in the thinking of these stake-holders.

---

[6] We are not arguing here in favour of a permissive approach to the use of banned substances as Cashmore (2003) has elsewhere [35]. His argument is essentially that the testing for banned substances is "expensive, ineffective, futile and a denial of the reality of contemporary sport". Except for a pedagogic purpose in the spirit of 'playing devil's advocate', this is not a view that we would advance.

[7] For instance, it might be possible to infer from the narratives something about Anya's greater sense of corporeality as a senior level competitor, Nick's paternalism as a coach, or Lionel's attitude to 'drink-driving'. None of these is intended.

2. The contemporary context of elite sport makes the possible benefits that accrue from success very attractive. It is a cliché, but fame and fortune are potentially powerful temptations – it has become a cliché because it is a truism.

3. There are differences within this sport regarding awareness of the use of banned substances. There is a gendered dimension (with the issues talked about less amongst women and girls), as well as a factor related to the transition from junior to senior levels of competition – the latter linked more clearly to the extrinsic rewards for success.

4. Whether real or imagined, there is a perception that British competitors are subjected to more rigorous out-of-competition testing, and this creates a sense of 'unfairness' and some resentment.

This chapter is based on a single case-study sport, but it is not even a complete account of that sport. Moreover, superficially at least, there are differences in the participation patterns between, say, rowing and track and field athletics, just as there are different career opportunities in professional cycling and swimming. Two further directions for research are therefore required. First, a study of greater breadth to examine the extent to which the views expressed in this study are shared by others within the sport. Second, a more developed portfolio of case-studies to be developed to shed light on the ways in which the issues associated with the use of banned substances are understood in different sports[8].

ACKNOWLEDGMENTS

We are grateful to the participants who were so generous with their time and so open and forthright in their discussions with us, and to Matthew Fleming and Stewart Fleming for their comments on draft versions of the narratives. The shortcomings in the final product are, of course, our responsibility not theirs.

---

[8] We realise, of course, that in our attempts to protect the identity of the sport concerned and the anonymity of the participants, we have necessarily made it difficult (if not impossible) for other researchers to know which sport should be investigated to extend the scope of the analysis within the sport itself, and which other sports need to be examined to provide a fuller picture across sports. A simple answer is that any research that sheds further light on the use of banned substances in sport adds constructively to the developing body of knowledge.

AUTHOR NOTES

Alex McInch is a PhD student in the sociology of sport at the Cardiff School of Sport, Cardiff Metropolitan University. His research interests include contemporary qualitative methodologies and the ethics of research, both of which were covered in his Masters Degree thesis. This project was an autoethnographic exploration into illness and its impact on relational identity within sport. His other research interests include identity and social theory.

Scott Fleming is Director of Research and Professor of Sport and Leisure Studies at the Cardiff School of Sport, Cardiff Metropolitan University. He has a long standing interest in methods of enquiry and the ethics of social research. His most recent published work includes contributions to research on choking in elite golf, personal narrative and the ethics of disclosure, the 'enforcer' in elite level sport, and community sport development.

Anna Leyshon is a Lecturer in Physical Education and Pedagogy in the Cardiff School of Sport, Cardiff Metropolitan University. As a qualified and former practising PE teacher, her research has focused on the health, physical activity and well being of young people. Her PhD (completed in 2011) was funded by Sport Wales and focused on young people's leisure lifestyles and their engagement with the '5x60' extracurricular physical activity programme in secondary schools across Wales.

REFERENCES

[1] *The Guardian* (2011e). Tour de France 2011: Alexandr Kolobnev withdraws after positive test. 12th July. Accessed on 14th July 2011 from: *http://www.guardian*

[2] *The Guardian* (2011b). 'Role model' shot putter Mark Edwards given three-year doping ban. 9th June. Accessed on 14th July 2011 from: *http://www.guardian*

[3] *The Guardian* (2011d). Sri Lanka's Upul Tharanga banned for three months for doping violation. 24th June. Accessed on 14th July 2011 from: *http://www.guardian*

[4] *The Guardian* (2011a). Five Mexico internationals at Gold Cup test positive for clenbuterol. 9th June. Accessed on 14th July 2011 from: *http://www.guardian*

[5]   *The Guardian* (2011c). Rotherham's Nico Steenkamp banned for methylhexaneamine use. 1st April. Accessed on 14th July 2011 from: *http://www.guardian*

[6]   Cohen, S. (2002) *Folk Devils and Moral Panics - 30th Anniversary Edition.* London: Routledge. London: Routledge.

[7]   Dimeo, P. (2007). A History of Drug Use in Sport: 1876 – 1976. *Beyond Good and Evil.*

[8]   Dimeo, P. (2009). Ed., *Drugs, Alcohol and Sport - A Critical History.* London: Routledge.

[9]   Fourcoy, J.L (2010). Ed., *Pharmacology, Doping and Sports - A Scientific Guide for Athletes, Coaches, Physicians, Scientists and Administrators.* London: Routledge.

[10]   McNamee, M. and Møller, V. (2011). Eds., *Doping and Anti-Doping Policy in Sport Ethical, Legal and Social Perspectives.* London: Routledge.

[11]   Møller, V. (2009). *The Ethics of Doping and Anti-Doping - Redeeming the Soul of Sport?* London: Routledge.

[12]   Stewart, C., Lord, R., Wiltshire, G. and Fleming, S. (2010). 'Ease of movement and freedom of corporeal expression? Femininity, the body and leotards in trampoline gymnastics'. In D. Chatziefstathiou and L. Mansfield, L. (eds.) *Leisure Identities and Authenticity* (pp.63-76), Eastbourne: Leisure Studies Association.

[13]   Sparkes, A.C. (1992). 'The Paradigms Debate'. In A.Sparkes (ed.), *Research in Physical Education and Sport,* (pp. 9-60), London: Falmer Press.

[14]   Sparkes, A.C. (1994). 'Research paradigms in physical education: some brief comment on differences that make a difference', *British Journal of Physical Education,* vol. 14, 1, 11-16.

[15]   Denzin, N.K. and Lincoln, Y.S. (2000). *Handbook of Qualitative Research.* Thousand Oaks: Sage Publications Limited.

[16]   Sparkes, A. (2000). 'Autoethnography and narratives of self: Reflections on criteria in action'. *Sociology of Sport Journal*, vol. 17, 1, 21-41.

[17]   Holt, N.L. (2003). 'Representation, Legitimation and Autoethnography: an autoethnographic writing story', *International Journal of Qualitative Methods,* vol. 2, 1, 1-22.

[18]   Carless, D. and Sparkes, A.C. (2008). 'The physical activity experiences of men with serious mental illness: Three short stories', *Psychology of Sport and Exercise,* vol. 9, 2, 191-210.

[19] Barone, T. E. (2000). *Aesthetics, politics, and educational inquiry: Essays and examples.* New York: Peter Lang.

[20] Angrosino, M. (1998). *Opportunity house: Ethnographic stories of mental retardation.* Walnut Creek, CA: Alta Mira.

[21] Agar, M. (1995). 'Literary journalism as ethnography'. In J. Van Maanen (ed.), *Representation in ethnography* (pp. 112–129). London: Sage.

[22] Maykut, P. and Moorhouse, R. (1994*). Beginning Qualitative Research: a philosophic and practical guide,* London: Routledge.

[23] MacIntyre, A. (1985). *After virtue: A study in moral theory,* 2nd edition. London: Duckworth.

[24] Loland, S. (2001). Ed., *Fair play in sport - A moral norm system.* London: Routledge.

[25] Bloodworth, A. and McNamee, M. (2010) 'Clean Olympians? Doping and anti-doping: The views of talented young British athletes'*, International Journal of Drug Policy,* vol. 21, 4, 276-282.

[26] Mills, C.W. (1959). *The Sociological Imagination,* New York: Oxford University Press.

[27] Bredemeier, B.J. and Shields, D.L. (1995). *Character development and physical activity.* Leeds: Human Kinetics.

[28] Fleming, S. and McNamee, M. (2005) 'The ethics of corporate governance in public sector organizations: Theory and method', *Public Management Review,* Vol. 7, 1, 135-144.

[29] Cashmore, E. (2005) *Making sense of sports,* 4th edition. London: Routledge.

[30] Wood, G. (2011). Nicky Henderson tells vets' inquiry 'plenty' used banned drug. *The Guardian,* 15th February. Accessed on 14th July 2011 from: *http://www.guardian*

[31] Mellick, M. and Fleming, S. (2010). 'Personal Narrative and the Ethics of Disclosure: a case study from elite sport', *Qualitative Research,* vol. 10, 3, 299-314.

[32] Tsang, T. (2000). 'Let Me Tell You a Story: A Narrative Exploration of Identity in High Performance Sport', *Sociology of Sport Journal,* vol. 17, 1, 44-59.

[33] Hockey, J and Allen-Collinson, J (2007). 'Grasping the phenomenology of sporting bodies'. *International Review for the Sociology of Sport,* vol. 42, 2, 115-131.

[34] Allen-Collinson, J. and Hockey, J. (2009). 'The essence of sporting embodiment: Phenomenological analyses of the sporting body', *The*

International Journal of Interdisciplinary Social Sciences, vol. 4, 4, 71-81.

[35] Cashmore, E. (2003) 'Stop testing and legalise the lot'. *The Observer*, 26th October. Accessed on 14th July 2011 from: *http://www.guardian*

In: Perspectives on Anabolic Androgenic ....   ISBN: 978-1-62081-243-3
Editors: F. Grace and J. S. Baker   © 2012 Nova Science Publishers, Inc.

Chapter 7

ANABOLIC ANDROGENIC STEROIDS (AAS), DOPING AND ENHANCEMENT ETHICS

A. J. Bloodworth and M. J. McNamee
Philosophy, Humanities and Law in Healthcare, College of Human
and Health Sciences, Swansea University, Swansea, Wales, UK

ABSTRACT

The aim of this chapter is to offer a consideration of philosophical
and ethical arguments that are grounded in the contexts of anabolic
androgenic steroid (AAS) use and doping in sports participation.

Sports may be seen as an unusual family of social practices that,
while aiming at excellence, delimits the legitimate ways in which
participants may prepare for, and perform in, those social practices.

The present chapter sketches the terrain within the academic
bioethics literature concerning the use of AAS for therapy and
enhancement.

There is examination as to the extent of the prevalence of AAS use
within the sporting environment including the standard arguments that are
raised within the philosophy of sports ethics giving consideration to the
specific policy position of the World Anti Doping Agency (WADA).

INTRODUCTION

The use of medical means to enhance human performance has been the subject of significant ethical interest [1;2]. The athletes and coaches engaged in elite sport are necessarily concerned with, indeed focused on, ways in which to maximise human performance. This makes sport an interesting arena within which to test intuitions regarding the value and permissibility of performance enhancing substances and technologies. Within the context of competitive sport, there is often dialogue concerning the use of banned performance enhancing drugs. In society, more broadly, performance enhancement for cognitive or cosmetic benefit has been the subject of debate. Exactly what constitutes enhancement, as opposed to having other medical procedures or therapies, is not as easy to define, as may be thought[1].

In an attempt to achieve some conceptual clarification, Tännsjö [3] offers a useful distinction between negative medical interventions, positive medical interventions and enhancements. Negative interventions aim at ameliorating, improving, or removing conditions of disease and disability; positive interventions aim at 'improving the functioning of an organism within a natural variation' [3]; enhancement aims at extending human functioning 'beyond the normal functioning of a human organism' [3] Tännsjö provides the examples of antibiotics to cure pneumonia as a negative medical intervention, human growth hormone being prescribed for an unusually small child as a positive medical intervention, and providing a man with 'big (female) breasts' [3] as an example of enhancement. Tännsjö further acknowledges that the current rules in sport appear to object to both positive medical interventions and enhancement.

The debate over the legitimacy of enhancements often utilises a contrast between therapy on the one hand, and enhancements on the other. There are some similarities with Tännsjö's line here. A therapeutic intervention seeks to treat a condition that has inhibited normal functioning. Such an intervention is concerned with restoring health often via the treatment of disease. Interventions intended to enhance are not concerned with restoration but with *elevation* beyond normal functioning or capacities, understood as "species-typical-functioning" [4]

The debate over the ethical desirability or defensibility of seeking to enhance our human capacities has been fiercely conducted in academic fields

---

[1] See Parens (1998) [1] for a complex philosophical analysis of the therapy / enhancement distinction.

and public media. Those supporting enhancements have sought to discredit distinctions such as those made between therapy and enhancement, or criticised concepts such as normal functioning, in order to demonstrate how enhancements are not ethically dissimilar from commonly accepted medical practice.

Examples of enhancing human capacities via medical, or more generally biotechnological, means are present within the sporting arena, but the debate extends beyond sport. Recent research in neuroethics has suggested significant use of cognitive enhancement by academics [5] and argued that it is a positive and desirable trend [6]. Equally the widespread use of Viagra suggests that "performance enhancement" is not restricted to sports domains. Enhancement of our physical appearance via medical means also appears to be a growing attraction, either via cosmetic surgery, or the use of substances to help attain a muscular, lean, or simply more sexualised physique.

The arguments that oppose the use of medical means to enhance human capabilities are often general in nature; they are not confined to a specific domain or type of enhancement [7]. Leon Kass, former chair of the US President's Bioethics Committee, and edited the widely cited biotechnologically conservative report "Beyond Therapy" [8] advances just such a general argument.

For Kass [9] a good life is one in which we can feel responsible for our achievements. He speaks of 'the merit of disciplined and dedicated striving' [9]. A flourishing life requires this effort and striving for what is valuable. However, taking banned substances for athletic or cognitive performance is not commensurable with this conception of a good life.

While Kass is concerned with all forms of medical enhancement, whether taken by the professor keen to publish or the athlete keen to run faster or train harder, there is evidence that this line of arguments resonates with young athletes. Qualitative research [10] has reported on athletes' concern with natural performance, being able to attribute achievement directly to the result of hard work and the guilt that would be associated with success having doped.

Having sketched out the bioethical context of debates concerning medical and biotechnological enhancement, the following section examines the prevalence of AAS (and related products) usage within a broader context of performance enhancements in sports.

PREVALENCE OF AAS AND PERFORMANCE ENHANCING DRUGS

Prior to considering the relative merits of ethical arguments, the prevalence of performance enhancing drug use will be considered. This is again a contentious issue, the extent to which banned substances are being utilised by elite athletes is difficult to determine. WADA reports low numbers of athletes testing positive for a banned substances (2% or lower) [11]. However, estimates of prevalence derived from athlete surveys, as opposed to actual test results have occasionally been as high as 20% [12].[2] While the actual extent of doping in sport is disputed, WADA's requirement that athletes are available for randomised testing throughout the year provides an indication of the perceived pervasiveness of the problem.

The use of doping substances such as anabolic-androgenic steroids for example, is not confined to athletes trying to gain a competitive advantage. In adults, anti-doping bodies report the use of such substances by those not involved in competitive sport. In 2009, Bojsen-Moller and Christiansen [13] analysed enquiries made to the Danish Anti-Doping Agency over an 18 month period. 1398 queries were examined. The service was found to be used in the main by males in their mid 20s, who were training in gymnasiums. Enquiries by those in competitive sports were sparse with enquiries from those engaged in elite sport even less. 15% of enquirers reported current or previous use of WADA banned substances, the majority (62%) citing AAS consumption.

Another Scandinavian study [14] sought to examine via qualitative means the background and story of those engaged in AAS use. The paper again notes that such substances are commonly used outside of athletic populations interested in appearance enhancement. The study sought to explore via 6 case studies, the development of AAS and other drug use in patients attending an addiction clinic in Sweden. Their attendance was motivated by current AAS use. Each user began AAS use alongside training at a gymnasium; onset of use was mostly in the late teens. Multiple drug use often followed, either to further stimulate gains in training, or to combat side-effects from AAS use.

---

[2] This study with German athletes employed a randomised response technique comprised of one question, basically have you ever used doping substances? (Or a variation such as have you in this season?), with an additional instruction. The additional instruction required athletes born in the months January to April to answer yes, and those born in other months to answer honestly. Thus even the researchers could not judge whether the individual athlete had taken performance enhancing drugs in this online survey, but calculated prevalence figures from the 'yes' and 'no' responses, and data concerning the frequency of births from January to April.

Motivation for use often concerned a perceived plateau in performance by natural means where AAS use offered an opportunity to overcome this. While initially positive effects of AAS use were reported – often associated with perceived attractiveness and social status, perceived positive effects were increasingly outweighed by the negative effects such as increased aggressiveness.

The onset of steroid use in teens, and indeed the possibility of a doping problem existing in our young people has been the topic of some research. Review studies (albeit predominantly North American) suggest between 3 and 12 % of adolescent males [15,16] have reported using AAS at some point. Use by females is reported to be lower, around 1-2% admitting using steroids [15]. Again, these data are not confined to participants in competitive sports. Of adolescents who reported using AAS, review articles suggest between 30 and 40 per cent were not engaged in competitive sport [15,16]. Among non-sporting motivations, the desire to increase muscle mass to enhance physical appearance is a dominant one [17].

Kanayama and coworkers (2007) [18] question these prevalence rates. Particularly concerned with prevalence in teenage girls they cite problems with the methodology of questionnaires, suggesting survey questions may have elicited false positive responses. For example, among those surveys that reported higher prevalence rates, questions failed to distinguish between anabolic steroids, corticosteroids, and other supplements that could be obtained over the counter, and the authors suggest, might be confused with steroids. They conclude that AAS use among teenage girls has been greatly overestimated, actual prevalence being as low as 0.1%. This contention is also applied to male prevalence, questionnaires deemed more reliable finding lower rates of around 1% or less (in those aged 14-19 years). In 2010, Harmer [19] further cites the possibility for inflated prevalence assessments stemming from flawed methodology. In this review Harmer suggests that use of AAS, rather than being connected to sport participation is more likely to be associated with broader problem behaviours, deviant behaviours and dissatisfaction with body image.

This suggestion that teen use of substances such as AAS is part of a wider tendency toward 'sensation seeking' behaviour has received some support. Dunn and White [20] surveyed reports on data gathered from 21905 students in Australian secondary schools aged 12-17 years who completed a questionnaire. 2.4% of students reported AAS use at some point. Use being more common among 12-15 year olds than 16-17 year olds. The factors associated with AAS use (both over a lifetime and in the past year) were being male, not being at school on the previous day, using a language other than English at home and rating your own academic ability as below average. The findings also suggested an association between AAS use and other substance use. Buckman and colleagues [21] also found that male college athletes who used performance enhancing substances were also more likely to use other drugs, and use alcohol in a problematic fashion. Those who used performance enhancing substances had higher 'sensation seeking' scores and were also more likely to have used tobacco, marijuana, cocaine, psychedelics, and prescription drugs without prescription during the previous year.

Dodge and Hoagland [22] also recently reviewed the relationship between AAS use and the use of other drugs. The majority of studies utilised adolescent samples from high schools or college. 56% of the studies were conducted in the U.S.A. All but one of the studies was cross-sectional. AAS use was found to be positively associated with the use of alcohol, illicit drugs and legal performance enhancing supplements. Studies found AAS use to be related to recent and overall alcohol use, as well as more problematic types of alcohol consumption for example binge drinking or harmful/problem drinking. The authors, however, recommend that more studies be done to ascertain the relationship between AAS use and particular types of drinking behaviour. The review makes a key observation, however, that the majority of studies measured AAS use in such a fashion as to reflect experimental use. Those experimenting with AAS were also more likely to experiment with other substances. Thus any possible relationship between habitual AAS use and other substance use is under researched and unexplained at present.

With regard to poly drug use, there is clear evidence in the studies of adult gym attendees in Wales, that multiple drugs are used, including but not limited to ephedrine, growth hormone, and substances taken to minimise the side effects of AAS consumption [23,24]. That adolescents using AAS are 'poly-drug users' [25], *and* these drugs extend to those not associated with improving performance or appearance appears to reflect a particular type of substance use. A sensation seeker experimenting with a range of substances. While we have reviewed evidence that supports such a profile in young people, there is evidence that older habitual users of AAS have a more functional view of their role. Monaghan (2002) reports on a sample with an average of 30, the majority being bodybuilders, sharply distinguishing between AAS use and the use of recreational drugs [26]. They abstained from recreational drug use, and in some cases alcohol, as they pursued their body ideal.

This tour of some selected literature paints a somewhat ambiguous picture. It is evident that AAS and similar compounds are being used both inside and outside of sport. Rates of prevalence are contested. WADA test results are often considered to be an underestimate, while suggestions of adolescent and female use my be overestimated. Motivations for such use may be functional, to achieve a particular body ideal or desired level of performance, or reflect adolescent experimentation. But to what extent should we be concerned with such use? As is clear from the resources directed toward anti-doping initiatives, there seems a prominent view among sports administrators that the use of performance enhancing substances conflicts with a sporting ethos.

ETHICAL AND PHILOSOPHICAL ARGUMENTS

Arguments such as those of Kass [8,9], which focus on the centrality of instrumental values such as struggling, striving and discipline, reflect a particular conception of the good life; a meritocratic one where talent and effort determine success. He argues that enhancing human performance via medical means is not a shortcut to a flourishing and fulfilling life, but actually takes us farther away from one. Within sports, the philosophy behind the ban on certain performance enhancing substances and techniques also utilises a particular substantive conception of what *sport* should be and the values it should reflect.

Some may conceive that the prohibition of AAS and other doping products as paradoxical in a society where pharmacologies are widespread: where there is (as the saying goes) a pill for every ill, and an ill for every pill. What are the standard arguments raised by philosophers with respect to doping use? It should be noted that most philosophers of sport that have published in academic literature are somewhat sceptical about the ethical basis for a ban on performance enhancing products. While the present authors (and editors) are supportive of the general anti-doping stance, the following offers an outline of the philosophical and ethical arguments for and against[3]. These may be summarised as follows: (i) that doping is all about performance enhancement; (ii) that doping allows an increased quality and quantity of training; (iii) that doping is unnatural; (iv) that doping is coercive; (iv) that doping is harmful; (v) that doping confers an unfair advantage.

---

[3] These summaries are adapted from McNamee (2008) [43].

(i) Doping is Wrong because it Enhances Performance

The weakest of all anti-doping arguments is oddly enough one that is commonly proposed in sports bars and cafés. It is that doping is wrong because it enhances performance. The position is straightforward but is open to two types of instant rebuttal. In the first instance one might ask whether it is indeed true that the banned substances we see on lists of prohibitions are indeed performance enhancing. Among others, Nicholson [27] nearly a quarter of a century ago claimed that the evidence was far from clear. Much of their performance enhancing effect, he suggests, is down to a placebo effect. It would be fair to say that the body of sports scientists would argue that he is wrong as a matter of fact. It may well be true, however, that we are not, or at least not always, in a position to identify clear cut explanations for enhanced performance that are caused by the doping substance or process while ignoring placebo effects. To the contrary, however, sporting excellence – doped or otherwise – will always be a complex product of human heart and mind, as much as extreme bodily efforts. A second, less easily dismissed, aspect of this argument refers to the very possibility of gathering such information. If one suspected x, y or z substances were performance enhancing but also likely to cause harm, how would one proceed to gain ethical approval for the research which tried to demonstrate such? So, it is said, the very idea of gaining a large and reliable inventory of doping products would be scuppered at the first stage by the inability to gain research ethics approval by the relevant regulating authority. Since the time these arguments were first raised, largely in the late 1980s, empirical work on performance enhancing products and substances has indeed emerged despite the scepticism of research ethics approval ever being granted to gain sufficiently large and reliable data. Recent UK studies of bodybuilding cultures both medical [24] and sociological [26] offer clear evidence of risks outside healthcare and medically related doping abuse.

(ii) Doping Allows an Increased Quality and Quantity of Training

In any event, it has been said by the skeptic, elite sports is all about enhancement, why worry specifically about pharmacological modes of enhancement. All elite competitors, and very many more mundane ones, push themselves to their limits looking for that extra degree of concentration, effort, speed, strength, or whichever capacity is prized in the various sports under discussion. One response to this problem is the idea that doping is wrong because, it is said, it allows some athletes to train harder than those who do not.

In many spheres we admire those who achieve distinction. Ought we to find ethically problematic athletes who dope in order to work harder? One may be on a caffeine-induced high as one reads this chapter late at night. Who would worry about that? A great many comedians and musicians are well known to suffer from a host of psychological deficiencies and can only face the audience when bolstered by alcohol or other drugs. Why should steroid use (or more generally any chemical or pharmaceutical means) to enhance sporting performance provoke our ire? Moreover, access to new facilities, higher levels of specialised coaching, increased nutritional sophistication and equipment technology (such as isokinetic resistance machines or hyperbaric chambers) all improve training effects without much controversy? We encourage other training enhancement methods, it is said, why not pharmacological enhancement?

One direct attack on pharmacological enhancement is the claim that doping is wrong because it is unnatural. Precisely what is natural is itself problematic. Nevertheless, even on the grounds of consistency it can be asked why approved substances and procedures such as sleeping in oxygen-deprived tents or chamber is thought to be any more 'natural'?[28;29;30;31;32].

Another feature of this move hat is open to attack is the idea that sports itself is not natural but an artifice: a social construction and institutionalisation of the impulse to play. So why then should we be worried about doping as unnatural? What ethical leverage is supposed to apply? If it is some unstated assumption that that which is natural is good and that which is unnatural is bad then one has only to wave that logical sword, the naturalistic fallacy, at such proponents. The naturalistic fallacy, in brief, holds that one may not move directly from statements of fact (what is the case) directly to moral conclusions (what ought to be). This is the move that is illicitly made between the jump that our natural bodies are good because they are natural, but unnatural ones are bad because they are unnatural (or analogously that natural performances are good and non-natural/artificially ones bad). And of course the conclusion *might* make for some indefensible positions on those with artificial limbs or replacement joints who (apparently) fall below the limit of what a natural body constitutes. It is reasonable to suppose that those who naively put forward the naturalistic argument have failed to consider the implications for such people who engage in sports in both able bodied and disability sports. The idea that an athlete with prostheses is somehow morally inferior to natural athletes (which is the consequence of the view) is deeply offensive to our modern egalitarian ideals. This raises in particular the issues of prosthetically enhanced athletes versus non-prosthetically enhanced performances [33] which, though interesting, lies beyond the scope of this chapter.

And yet, there is something in the view that our human nature deserves respect which is not fully articulated in this view of the unnaturalness of doping whether pharmacological or genetic. As Miah [34] points out, part of it is objection is an irrational fear of some kind of mythical Frankenstein. Miah is correct to be wary of the unscrupulous or manipulative deployment of the concept, "natural", (which is open to interpretation) but there is no reason to think that the normative utilisation of naturalness in arguments against doping lead us necessarily to condemn or disvalue disabled populations who rely on artificial or technological products in their daily living. Notwithstanding all this, the idea of a non-natural body enhanced from our ideas of normal human functioning is one that troubles many philosophers and scientists alike.[4]

(iii) Doping is Coercive

It is sometimes said by athletes themselves, that doping-related bans are justified to prevent their coercion into taking drugs. Or, as Ben Johnson's coach, Charlie Francis, famously put it: 'if you don't take it you won't make it'. Allowing athletes to dope may coerce other athletes into participating in an AAS using regimen against their will. There is a close relationship between the apparent coercion argument and the train-harder argument. When a colleague eschews the model of a family life and, like a hermit, works twelve hours a day, 5 days a week, and 50 weeks a year we may just as easily admire their industry as we may mock their lack of balance. Would we have grounds for saying, at the next promotion board, that the promotion ought not go to the super-industrious on the grounds that their work habits have a coercive effect on all those who wish to achieve the said promotion in the future? Not every social pressure may count as a coercive one. But if coercion means something like the wrongful restriction of an agent's freedom then we would be hard pressed to locate our fellow, dope-driven, athletes the ascription 'coercers'. In what sense are they coercing their opponents? Can athletes not simply choose a dope-free option to training and performance? Is it not, rather, that a free choice not to participate, or to participate in legal and legitimate ways, is still

---

[4] Though not all of course. See, for example, Miah (2004)[34] and Savulescu et al. (2007) [38].

possible. We do not say to our gut-busting colleague that they ought to be prevented from accessing their workstation, or the library, or their personal computers after so many hours. We respect their autonomy even if we deride the narrowness of their industriousness. And on a point of consistency, if our arguments were truly about the concern that others inflicted upon us, that should apply to all practices such as athletes who run for more miles or in higher climates, swimmers who do more lengths, cross-country skiers who sleep in so-called oxygen tents to boost their production of red blood cells and improve oxygen transportation around the body. What about cyclists who wear aerodynamic hats, swimmers who wear fast-skin suits, or female gymnasts who are forced to discipline their bodies by calorific control to achieve outrageous morphological norms which are inappropriate for certain ages and body types and often deeply corrosive to their psychological well-being. What about jockeys who are 'coerced' to "waste" (to lose weight by the excessive use of fasting, saunas, and often smoking) to achieve the weight that horse trainer believes is optimum for his or her thoroughbred?.

(iv) Doping is Harmful

The coercion argument is itself related to a more general justification of doping bans (and *mutatis mutandis* other allegedly unethical practices that are made impermissible by the rules), that of preventing harm to athletes. Doping substances it is claimed are harmful to the athletes concerned. As noted above, there is a degree of consensus that some doping substances and processes are harmful, not all banned substances are harmful or at least not necessarily harmful. Might the blood doping under supervised medical conditions provide such a model? (though certainly a more respectful version of the East German doping scandals of the seventies and eighties).

If it were true that all doping products and substances were harmful, there would need to be a fielding of questions as to why one should feel bad faith towards the ranges of harms associated with doping, as opposed to our benign acceptance towards combat sports, such as boxing, where harm is intrinsic to the activity. What about the deaths from equestrian sports, of horse and rider alike? What about the number of paraplegics whose disability has been caused from forceful contact with the ground and with other players in rugby and American football? Less dramatically, what about the legion of football players around the world with arthritic ankles, hips and knees. Can we discount the magnitude of harm here?

As with the range of other practices that might be thought impermissible in the discussion on coercion, we find ourselves confronted with the question 'what are the limits on "paternalistic interference" in sport?' Finding a satisfactory answer to this question ought properly to precede banning doping it might reasonably be said.

(v) Doping Confers an Unfair Advantage

Perhaps the most commonly discussed criterion in support of anti-doping protocol has been the argument that it represents an unfair advantage to those who attempt to subvert the rules of sport. Let us assume that the bans are based on the efficacy of the substances and processes so included. In this way we can set aside the fact that advantage does accrue to the doped athlete. The standard position against the unfairness argument is the skeptical one of inconsistency: unfair advantages abound in sport. Examples spring readily to mind. What should we say of athletes born in high altitude who develop greater oxygen carrying capacities? What about those born in wealthier nations who can rely on sophisticated technological systems support? What about teams that are sponsored by multi-national companies or wealthy businessmen compared to relatively impoverished opponents?

These summaries merely point to the complex arguments that philosophers have traded in the war of words concerning (il)licit performance enhancement in sports. Nevertheless, it is important to distinguish general philosophical arguments from the policies of national and international sports bodies and in particular those of the World Anti Doping Agency (WADA) [35], who set global standards for the proscription of doping.

OFFICIAL RESPONSES TO STEROID DERIVED PERFORMANCE ENHANCMENT IN SPORTS: WADA'S POSITION

WADA have, with global support of state's parties, generated a list of prohibited substances, those that's use contravene the rules of the sporting contest and will result in sanction of some kind. The World Anti Doping Code (WADC) [35] considers whether or not to ban a substance on the basis of its fulfilling two of the following three criteria: that it (i) enhances or has the potential to enhance performance (ii) threatens health or has the potential to do so; and (iii) is 'contrary to the spirit of sport' [11] or by acting as a masking agent in relation to a prohibited substance.

This ban on certain substances or methods, however, has been the subject of strong critique. That the 'spirit of sport' be used as part of the criteria has lead to claims that such a notion is not operationalisable in policy terms [36, 37] It has also been claimed that rather then being contrary to the spirit of sport, using medical means to directly change our biology reflects this spirit and indeed the human spirit more generally.

> We can choose what kind of competitor to be, not just through training, but through biological manipulation. Human sport is different from animal sport because it is creative. Far from being against the spirit of sport, biological manipulation embodies the human spirit—the capacity to improve ourselves on the basis of reason and judgment. When we exercise our reason, we do what only humans do [38].

As we have seen, it has also been suggested that the ban of performance enhancing substances on health grounds is essentially hypocritical. Elite sport, it is argued, is an inherently unhealthy activity [36, 39]. The growing cost of administering anti-doping programmes [40] and the infringement upon athlete privacy of year round random drugs testing [32, 41] have also been raised in order to undermine the legitimacy of the WADA ban.

The prohibition of performance enhancing substances, it has been argued, is more harmful in the long term. Athletes with solely the potential gains in performance in mind are thought to utilise banned substances without considering their health [39]. An alternative would be to test for levels of substances, rather than ban the substances altogether [38]. It is suggested that in this kind of 'open-doping' athletes would be monitored for levels of substances and if tests indicated an unhealthy or dangerous level they would be excluded on these grounds [38]. This debate also concerns the limits of paternalistic action. Can the present ban on performance enhancing substances be justified as an act designed to preserve the best interests of competitors? Or, in light of apparent inconsistencies, such as the general harms to health associated with many elite sports, should we at least enable greater choice for the athlete by permitting doping within certain limits set by discernable levels of danger? Open-doping, it might be suggested properly respects the autonomy of the competitor. The rationale behind such an approach might make clear that elite sport entails certain harms to health associated with training, competition, and perhaps even the range of technologies and supplements used. It suggests however, a certain limit to the sorts of harms that are acceptable by testing for 'safe' levels of substances. In an open environment the contraindications of doping substances may come to the fore, and athletes will be able to make an informed choice as to whether to dope within certain restrictions. Others have urged caution, however arguing that open-doping may not necessarily result in the safer use of such substances. Holm [42] contends that open-doping within safe parameters would only occur for the use of substances which all athletes are already aware of. In an instance where a new method or doping substance becomes available athletes would only be able to retain the competitive advantage by taking the substance, but keeping it secret. In instances where an athlete keeps a new substance secret, careful monitoring of the drug and side effects would be prevented.

CONCLUSION

Sports are conservative social practices that celebrate meritocratic principles of fairly rewarding hard work and talent. This is the thesis to support certain pharmacological prohibitions upon preparation and participation in competitive sport. The present chapter outlined the philosophical argument surrounding the impact of AAS and related compounds on the continued ethical debate on the use of pharmacological agents in the context of sports participation. Sustained and complex argument and policy are unlikely to be settled in the near, or for that matter not-so-near, future.

REFERENCES

[1]   Parens, E. (1998). Is Better Always Good?, In: Parens, E. (Ed.) *Enhancing Human Traits: Ethical and Social Implications*, (pp. 1-28) Washington DC: Georgetown University Press.
[2]   Rajczi, A. (2008). One Danger of Biomedical Enhancements, *Bioethics*, 22(6): 328-336.
[3]   Tännsjö, T. (2009). Medical Enhancement and the ethos of elite sport, In: Savulescu, J. & Bostrom, N. (Eds.) *Human Enhancement*, (pp. 315-326) Oxford: Oxford University Press.

[4]   Boorse, C. (1977). Health as a Theoretical Concept, *Philosophy of Science* 44: 542-73.

[5]   Sahakian, B. and Morein-Zamir, S. (2007) 'Professor's little helper', *Nature*, 450, 1157-1159.

[6]   Greely, H., Sahakian B., Harris J., Kessler R.C., Gazzaniga M., Campbell P. & Farah, M.J. (2008). Towards responsible use of cognitive-enhancing drugs by the healthy, *Nature*, 456, 702-705.

[7]   Douglas, T.M. (2007). Enhancement in Sport, and Enhancement outside Sport, *Studies in Ethics, Law, and Technology*, Volume 1, Issue 1 Article 2. DOI: 10.2202/1941-6008.1000.

[8]   Kass, L.R. & President's Council on Bioethics (2003a). *Beyond Therapy: Biotechnology and the Pursuit of Happiness a Report by the President's Council on Bioethics*, New York: Harper Collins

[9]   Kass, L.R. (2003b). Ageless Bodies, Happy Souls: Biotechnology and the Pursuit of Perfection, *The New Atlantis*, Spring: 9-28.

[10] Bloodworth, A.J. and McNamee, M.J. (2009). Clean Olympians? Doping and anti-doping: The views of talented young British athletes, *International Journal of Drug Policy*, 21: 276-282.

[11] [World Anti Doping Association (WADA). Annual Reports between 2002 – 2009 Available Online. *<http://www.wada-ama.org/en/Resources/Publications/Annual-Report/>* Accessed 20 June 2011.

[12] Pitsch, W., Emrich, E., Klein, M. (2005). Zur Häufigkeit des Dopings im Leistungssport: Ergebnisse eines www-surveys. [Doping in elite sports in Germany: results of a www survey] *Leipziger Sportwissenschaftliche Beiträge*, 46: 63-77.

[13] Bojsen-Moller, J. and Christiansen, A.V. (2010). Use of performance- and image-enhancing substances among recreational athletes: a quantitative analysis of inquiries submitted to the Danish anti-doping authorities, *Scandinavian Journal of Medicine and Science in Sports*, 20: 861-867.

[14] Skårberg, K., Nyberg, F., Engström, I. (2008). The development of multiple drug use among anabolic-androgenic steroid users: six subjective case reports, *Substance Abuse Treatment, Prevention, and Policy*, 3: 24 doi: 10.1186/1747-597X-3-24.

[15] Yesalis, C.E. and Bahrke, M.S. (2000). Doping among adolescent athletes. *Baillière's Clinical Endocrinology and Metabolism*, 14(1), 25-35.

[16] Calfee, R. and Fadale, P. (2006). Popular Ergogenic Drugs and Supplements in Young Athletes, *Pediatrics,* 117(3), e577-e589.

[17] Field, A.E., Bryn Austin, S., Camargo, C.A., Barr Taylor, C., Striegel-Moore, R.H., Loud, K. J., and Colditz, G.A. (2005). Exposure to the Mass Media, Body Shape Concerns, and the Use of Supplements to Improve Weight and Shape Among Male and Female Adolescents, *Pediatrics*, 116(2): e214-e220.

[18] Kanayama, G., Boynes, M., Hudson, J.I., Field, A.E., Pope Jr, H.G. (2007). Anabolic steroid abuse among teenage girls: An illusory problem? *Drug and Alcohol Dependence*, 88: 156-162.

[19] Harmer, P.A. (2010). Anabolic-androgenic steroid use among young male and female athletes: is the game to blame? *British Journal of Sports Medicine*, 44: 26-31

[20] Dunn, M. and White, V. (2011). The epidemiology of anabolic-androgenic steroid use among Australian secondary school students *Journal of Science and Medicine in Sport*, 14: 10-14.

[21] Buckman, J.F., Yusko, D.A., White, H.R., Pandina, R.J. (2009). Risk profile of male college athletes who use performance enhancing substances, *Journal of Studies on Alcohol and Drugs*, 919- 923.

[22] Dodge, T., and Hoagland, M.F. (2011). The use of anabolic androgenic steroids and polypharmacy: A review of the literature, *Drug and Alcohol Dependence*, 114:100-109.

[23] Baker, J.S., Graham, M.R. and Davies, B. (2006). Steroid and prescription medicine abuse in the health and fitness community: A regional study, *European Journal of Internal Medicine*, 17: 479-484.

[24] Grace, F., Baker, J. and Davies, B. (2001). Anabolic androgenic steroid use in recreational gym users: a regional sample of the mid Glamorgan area, *Journal of Substance Use*, 6: 189-195.

[25] Bahrke, M.S., Yesalis, C.E., Kopstein, A.N. and Stephens, J.A. (2000). Risk Factors Associated with Anabolic Androgenic Steroid Use Among Adolescents, *Sports Medicine,* 29(6), 397-405.

[26] Monaghan, L.F. (2002). Vocabularies of motive for illicit steroid use among bodybuilders, *Social Science and Medicine*, 55: 695-708.

[27] Nicholson, R. (1987). Drugs in sport; a reappraisal. *Institute of Medical Ethics Bulletin,* (Suppl.) 7:1-25.

[28] Fricker, P. (2005). Commentary: hypoxic air machines: *Journal of Medical Ethics*, 31: 115.

[29] Loland S. and Murray T.H. (2007). The ethics of the use of technologically constructed high-altitude environments to enhance

performances in sport, *Scandinavian Journal of Medicine and Science in Sports*, 17: 193-197.

[30] Spriggs, M. (2005). Hypoxic air machines: performance enhancement through effective training – or cheating?, *Journal of Medical Ethics*, 31: 112-13.

[31] Tamburrini, C. (2005). Commentary: hypoxic air machines, *Journal of Medical Ethics*, 31: 114.

[32] Tännsjö, T. (2005). Commentary: hypoxic air machines, *Journal of Medical Ethics*, 31: 113.

[33] Burkett, B., McNamee, M.J. and Potthast, W. (2012 *in press*). Shifting boundaries in sports technology and disability, is this equal rights or unfair advantage? A multidisciplinary analysis of Oscar Pistorius' Olympic Games eligibility' *Disability and Society*, 26(5).

[34] Miah, A. (2004). *Genetically modified athletes*, Abingdon: Routledge.

[35] World Anti Doping Association (WADA). World Anti-Doping Code. (2009). Available Online <http://www.wada-ama.org/en/World-Anti-Doping-Program/Sports-and-Anti-Doping-Organizations/The-Code/>. Accessed online 20 June 2011.

[36] Foddy, B. and Savulescu, J. (2007). Ethics of performance enhancement in sport: drugs and gene doping, In: Ashcroft, R.E., Dawson, R., Draper, H., McMillan, J. (Eds.) *Principles of healthcare ethics*, 2nd edition (pp. 511-520) London: Wiley.

[37] Møller, V. (2009). *The Ethics of Doping and Anti-Doping*. Abingdon: Routledge.

[38] Savulescu, J., Foddy, B., and Clayton, M. (2004). Why we should allow performance enhancing drugs in sport; British Journal of Sports Medicine, 38: 666–670.

[39] Kayser B. and Smith, A.C.T. (2008) Globalisation of anti-doping: the reverse side of the medal, *British Medical Journal*, 337, a584.

[40] Lippi, G., Banfi, G., Franchini, M., Cesare Guidi, G. (2008). New strategies for doping control, *Journal of Sports Sciences*, 26(5): 441-45.

[41] Kreft, L. (2009). The Elite Athlete – In a State of Exception?, *Sport, Ethics and Philosophy*. 3(1), 3-18.

[42] Holm, S. (2007). Doping Under Medical Control: Conceptually Possible but Impossible in the World of Professional Sports, *Sport, Ethics and Philosophy*, 1(2): 135-145.

[43] McNamee, M.J. (2008). Anti anti-doping: why scepticism doesn't cut the mustard, *British Medical Journal*, 337: a584.

In: Perspectives on Anabolic Androgenic ....   ISBN: 978-1-62081-243-3
Editors: F. Grace and J. S. Baker   © 2012 Nova Science Publishers, Inc.

Chapter 8

CURRENT HORMONES IN USE FOR PERFORMANCE AND IMAGE ENHANCEMENT

Michael Graham[*,1]*, Peter Evans*[2] *and Bruce Davies*[3]

[1] Sport and Exercise Science, Institute of Health, Medical Science and
Society Science, Glyndwr University, Wrexham, Wales, UK
[2] Dept Diabetes & Endocrinology, Royal Gwent Hospital, Newport,
Gwent, Wales, UK
[3] Dept of Health & Exercise Science, University of Glamorgan,
Mid Glamorgan. Wales, UK

FOREWORD

At the time of going to press (December, 2011), the lawyers of Lance Armstrong, the highly decorated cyclist, prepare for a United States federal investigation into whether Armstrong took performance enhancing-drugs. In Switzerland, The Court of Arbitration for Sport is hearing the case of alleged doping by Alberto Contador, the 2010 Tour de France winner. If, at worst, both were to be found guilty, then 14 of the past 16 winners of the Tour de France will have been doping for performance enhancement.

---

*Sport and Exercise Science, Institute of Health, Medical Science and Society Science, Glyndwr
University, Wrexham, Wales, UNITED KINGDOM, LL11 2AW. email: m.graham@
glyndwr.ac.uk.

ABSTRACT

Athletes are taking growth hormone and insulin, separately or in combination with the intention of increasing skeletal muscle mass hoping to improve performance and there is powerful scientific evidence to suggest this is possible. Adding some insulin-like growth factor, for example, Epo and myostatin inhibitor to the mixture and an almost undetectable cocktail is created that can promote significant muscle growth. Each of these drugs is on the World Anti-Doping Agency's (WADA's) banned list. However, if they are cycled correctly and unless an athlete is caught in possession of the drugs or tested within 24 hours of administration, the opportunity of proving a case of doping diminishes exponentially. There appears to be little problem obtaining such agents. These elixirs are not for sale from local superstores, but from unlicensed laboratories, to which the Internet has given *bona fide* credibility and a medium for conveyance.

INTRODUCTION

Since the isolation of human growth hormone (GH) in 1945 [1], and the synthesis of recombinant human growth hormone (rhGH) by recombinant DNA technology in the mid 1980s [2], strong anecdotal evidence suggests that athletes have been trying to extrapolate the proven benefits of replacement therapy in GH deficiency (GHD) to achieve supremacy, in the ultimate competition; the Olympics [3].

Strong anecdotal evidence exists that they are taking rhGH, recombinant human insulin-like growth factor (rhIGF) and insulin, separately or in combination, as doping agents to fulfil their dreams [4]. The use of and manipulation of testosterone and androgenic anabolic steroids (AAS) is "old hat"! What is not known is the extent of usage of other banned "designer-doping agents" being used to obtain the "ever-elusive" gold medal at the next Olympics.

Agents such as mechano growth factor (MGF), basic fibroblast growth factor (B-FGF), platelet derived growth factor (PDGF), vascular endothelial growth factor (VEGF), transforming growth factor b (TGF-b), bone morphogenetic protein (BMP) and leukaemia inhibitory factor (LIF) are growth factors (GFs) with the potential to cure injuries but are also of interest to athletes and may be powerful performance enhancers [5].

PREVALENCE AND PATTERNS OF GROWTH HORMONE AND INSULIN USE IN SPORT

Growth hormone (GH) appeared in the underground doping literature in 1981 [6]. An extensive literature research will identify very few cases of rhGH or insulin abuse by athletes. The few cases of rhGH abuse that have been published are case histories of individuals who have been arrested in possession at international tournaments. The possession of rhGH by the Chinese swimmers bound for the 1998 World Swimming Championships and similar problems at the Tour de France cycling event in 1998 suggested abuse at an elite level [7]. Approximately 1500 vials were stolen from an Australian wholesale chemist six months prior to the Sydney Olympics in 2000 [8]. The covert nature of its abuse precludes exact figures.

The few cases of insulin abuse that have been highlighted are those that have been admitted to hospital following accidental overdose [9;10]. In 2001, Dawson [11] reported that 10% of 450 patients attending his needle exchange programme, self-prescribe insulin for non-therapeutic purposes. A questionnaire survey by [12] has shown an increase in the abuse of insulin from 8%, to 14%, and an increase in the abuse of GH from 6%, to 24%, in comparison to a survey conducted by Grace and coworkers 2001 [13].

The first positive test for rhGH was on the former rugby league international Terry Newton in 2009 [14]. Newton confessed to the offence following A sample analysis and did not challenge the charge with analysis of his B sample. The second positive test was on the German cyclist Patrik Sinkewitz in 2011 [15]. However, due to the short window of opportunity of detection (<24 hours) such success in anti-doping remains a rarity.

Physiology of Growth Hormone

A cascade of interacting transcription factors and genetic elements normally determines the ability of the somatotroph cells in the anterior pituitary to synthesize and secrete the polypeptide human growth hormone (hGH). The development and proliferation of somatotrophs are largely determined by a gene called the Prophet of Pit-1 (PROP1), which controls the embryonic development of cells of the Pit-1 (POU1F1) transcription factor lineage. Pit-1 binds to the growth hormone promoter within the cell nucleus, a step that leads to the development and proliferation of somatotrophs and growth hormone transcription. Once translated, growth hormone is secreted as a 191-amino-acid, 4-helix bundle protein, weighing 22,000 daltons (70-80%) and a less abundant 176-amino-acid form, weighing 20,000 daltons (20-30%), [16;17] It enters the circulation in pulsatile fashion under dual hypothalamic control through hypothalamic-releasing and hypothalamic-inhibiting hormones that traverse the hypophysial portal system and act directly on specific somatotroph surface receptors [18].

Growth hormone releasing hormone (GHRH) induces the synthesis and secretion of growth hormone, and somatostatin suppresses the secretion of growth hormone. Growth hormone is also regulated by ghrelin, a growth hormone secretagogue–receptor ligand [19] that is synthesized mainly in the gastrointestinal tract. In healthy persons, the GH level is usually undetectable (<0.2 $\mu g.L^{-1}$) throughout most of the day. There are approximately 10 intermittent pulses of growth hormone per 24 hours, most often at night, when the level can be as high as 30 $\mu g.L^{-1}$ [18].

Fasting increases the secretion of growth hormone, whereas ageing and obesity are associated with suppressed secretory bursts of the hormone [20]. The action of growth hormone is mediated by a growth hormone receptor, which is expressed mainly in the liver and in cartilage and is composed of preformed dimers that undergo conformational change when occupied by a growth hormone ligand, promoting signalling [21]. Cleavage of the growth hormone receptor also yields a circulating growth hormone binding protein (GHBP), which prolongs the half-life and mediates the cellular transport of growth hormone. Growth hormone activates the growth hormone receptor, to which the intracellular Janus kinase 2 (JAK2) tyrosine kinase binds. Both the receptor and JAK2 protein are phosphorylated, and signal transducers and activators of transcription (STAT) proteins bind to this complex. STAT proteins are then phosphorylated and translocated to the nucleus, which initiates transcription of growth hormone target proteins [22].

Intracellular growth hormone signalling is suppressed by several proteins, especially the suppressors of cytokine signalling (SOCS). GH induces the synthesis of peripheral insulin-like growth factor-I (IGF-I) [23] and both circulating (endocrine) and local (autocrine and paracrine) IGF-I induces cell proliferation and inhibits apoptosis [24]. IGF-binding proteins (IGFBP) and their proteases regulate the access of ligands to the IGF-I receptor, either enhancing or attenuating the action of IGF-I. Levels of IGF-I are highest during late adolescence and decline throughout adulthood; these levels are determined by sex and genetic factors [25]. The production of IGF-I is suppressed in malnourished patients, as well as in patients with liver disease, hypothyroidism, or poorly controlled diabetes. IGF-I levels usually reflect the secretory activity of growth hormone and are one of a potential number of markers for identification of rhGH administration in sport [26].

In conjunction with GH, IGF-I has varying differential effects on protein, glucose, lipid and calcium metabolism [27] and therefore body composition. Direct effects result from the interaction of GH with its specific receptors on target cells. In the adipocyte, GH stimulates the cell to break down triglyceride and suppresses its ability to uptake and accumulate circulating lipids. Indirect effects are mediated primarily by IGF-I. Many of the growth promoting effects of GH, are due to the action of IGF-I on its target cells. In most tissues, IGF-I has local autocrine and paracrine actions, but the liver actively secretes IGF-I and its binding proteins, into the circulation. Our knowledge of the expression of skeletal muscle-specific isoforms of IGF-I gene in response to exercise in humans, is in its infancy.

Is rhGH the Anabolic Agent to Use in Sport?

Studies have demonstrated a decreased psychological well-being in hypopituitary patients, despite replacement with all hormones but GH [28]. An ergogenic aid is any external influences which can positively affect physical or mental performance. At the very least, winning any competition is, in part, "mental". In research, sports-persons have shown an improvement in psychological profile following rhGH administration [29]. Athletes have attempted to extrapolate this effect to the sporting arena.

The first researchers experimented on athletes using biosynthetic N-methionyl hGH (met-hGH), consisting of 192 amino-acids, as opposed to rhGH (191 amino acids). The administration of met-hGH (2.67 mg, three days per week) for six weeks in eight resistance-trained exercising adults, (aged 22-33 years) decreased body fat and increased lean body mass (LBM) [30]. Following the synthesis of rhGH and the benefits in GHD, early studies highlighted that an acute bolus administration in normal healthy humans in the post-absorptive state, was shown to increase net balance of forearm amino acids [31]. The major actions of GH are that it is a very potent anabolic agent, promoting protein synthesis and simultaneous lipolysis. These benefits are commonly acknowledged in sport. It stimulates protein synthesis through mobilisation of amino acid transporters in a similar manner to insulin and glucose transporters [8].

RhGH administration significantly increases the myosin heavy chain (MHC) 2X isoforms which the authors suggested was a change into a more youthful composition, possibly induced by the rejuvenation of systemic insulin-like growth factor-I (IGF-I) levels [32]. However, it had no effect on isokinetic quadriceps muscle strength, power, cross-sectional area (CSA), or fibre size. Resistance training (RT) and placebo, together, caused substantial increases in quadriceps isokinetic strength, power, and CSA, but these RT induced improvements were not further augmented by additional rhGH administration. In the RT and GH group, there was a significant decrease in MHC 1 and 2X isoforms, whereas MHC 2A increased. Healy and colleagues (2003) [33] identified that rhGH administered for 4 weeks in a dose of 0.067 mg.kg^{-1}.day^{-1}, to six males, exerted an anabolic effect both at rest and during exercise in endurance-trained athletes. Plasma levels of glycerol and free fatty acids (FFA) and glycerol rate of appearance (Ra) at rest, during and after exercise increased. Glucose Ra and glucose rate of disappearance (Rd) were greater after exercise, and resting energy expenditure and fat oxidation were greater under resting conditions. Acipimox is a niacin derivative and an anti-lipolytic. When administered with rhGH in a fasting state, it eliminated the ability of GH to restrict fasting protein loss. This indicated that stimulation of lipolysis by GH is its principle protein-conserving mechanism. Also muscle protein breakdown increased by 50% [34].

Ehrnborg et al., (2005) [35] administered rhGH for four weeks in a dose of 0.033 mg.kg^{-1}.day^{-1} and a dose of 0.067 mg.kg^{-1}.day^{-1} to a cohort of physically active individuals of both genders, with a mean age of 26 years. Despite no increase in strength being observed, IGF-I increased by 134%, body weight increased by 2.7%, LBM increased by 5.3% and body fat decreased by 6.6%.Plasma levels of glycerol and free fatty acids increased at rest and during exercise during rhGH administration, 0.067 mg.kg^{-1}.day^{-1}, for four weeks, in six trained male athletes. The resultant effect was an increase in both resting energy expenditure and fat oxidation, along with an increase in glucose production and uptake after exercise [36]. The results of these studies support the hypothesis of performance enhancement.

Myostatin is a transforming growth factor-β (TGF-β) family member that plays an essential role in regulating skeletal muscle growth. It acts as a negative regulator of skeletal muscle mass. Pharmacological agents capable of blocking myostatin activity may have applications for promoting muscle growth in human disease. Myostatin and messenger ribonucleic acid (mRNA) expression in the vastus lateralis, was significantly inhibited to 31% of controls during 18 months of treatment with rhGH in adult onset GHD. These effects were associated with significantly increased LBM and translated into significantly increased $\dot{V}$ O$_2$max [37]. Repetitive strain injuries can lead to stress fractures, tendonitis and possible tendon rupture. RhGH may prevent such injuries by the elevation of collagen and bone markers (osteocalcin, procollagen type III [P-III-P], type I collagen telopeptide [ICT] and C-terminal propeptide of type I collagen [PICP]) [38]. Correspondingly if injuries are present rhGH may enhance the healing process. Further research data would suggest that rhGH administration also has an effect on exercise performance [39]. The most conclusive results that supported performance enhancement were a series of studies [40]

Physical exercise may result in catabolism. Studies were conducted in a simulated catabolic state in sports-persons, with a mean age of 32 years. Catabolism was identified by baseline IGF-I levels being below 200 ng.ml^{-1}. A cohort of 24 males during the administration of rhGH, 0.019 mg.kg^{-1} day^{-1}, were compared with a cohort of 24 controls, for one week. Beneficial effects were achieved in psychological profile, strength (bench press and squat), aerobic power ($\dot{V}$ O$_2$max), respiratory function and anaerobic power (peak power output). In the optimum nutritional and training environment, rhGH may enhance constructive skeletal muscle development, to a supraphysiological status. This is a genuine belief determined from confessions from athletes, such as Ben Johnson, Kelly White, Tim Montgomery, Marion Jones and Dwain Chambers [41]. RhGH is currently undetectable by urinalysis. Detection is by blood analysis [42] but has yet to be subjected to legal challenge in court under the strictest scientific rigour [43]. A method of cycling the drug, one week on, one week off, can have significant effects on performance whilst thwarting the current detection techniques of the authorities [39].

Physiology of Insulin-Like Growth Factor-I (IGF-I)

The insulin-like growth factors (IGFs) are *proteins* with high *sequence similarity* to *insulin*. IGFs are part of a *complex system* that cells use to communicate with their environment. This complex system (often referred to as the IGF "axis") consists of two *cell-surface receptors* (IGF1R and IGF2R), two *ligands* (IGF-1 and IGF-2), a family of six high-affinity *IGF-binding proteins* (IGFBP 1-6), as well as associated *IGFBP* degrading *enzymes*, referred to collectively as *proteases. Insulin-like growth factor-1* (IGF-1) is mainly secreted by the liver and is induced by GH secretion [23]. Endocrine, autocrine and paracrine IGF-I induces cell proliferation and is thought to inhibit apoptosis [24].

IGF-1 consists of 70 amino acids in a single chain with three intramolecular disulfide bridges. IGF-1 has a molecular weight of 7649 daltons. It displays obvious homology to proinsulin, the precursor of insulin. Insulin like growth factor-I (IGF-I) mediates some of the metabolic actions of GH and has both GH-like and insulin-like actions. Both GH and IGF-I have a net anabolic effect enhancing whole body protein synthesis over a period of weeks, improving anthropometry in GHD. Both hormones have been used in catabolism and have been effective in counteracting the protein wasting effects of glucocorticoids. IGF-I administration improves insulin sensitivity, whereas GH therapy can be associated with compensatory hyperinsulinaemia.

Insulin-like growth (IGF-2) is thought to be a primary *growth factor* required for early development while *IGF-1* expression is required for achieving maximal growth. Factors that are known to cause variation in the levels of GH and IGF-1 in the circulation include genetic make-up, diurnal variation, age, sex, exercise status, stress levels, nutrition and disease state. IGF-1 has an involvement in regulating *neurogenesis, myelination, synaptogenesis*, and *dendritic* branching and *neuroprotection* after neuronal damage. IGFBPs and their proteases regulate the access of ligands to the IGF-1 receptor affecting its action. Levels of IGF-1 are at their peak during late adolescence and decline throughout adulthood, mirror imaging GH (Milani et al., 2004).The IGF-1 level reflects the secretory activity of growth hormone and is a marker for identification of GH-deficiency (GHD), or excess [44]. The concomitant administration of rhGH and rhIGF in GH resistant states has been shown to be synergistic and have effects that are far greater than either alone. Commercial pharmaceutical companies, e.g. Ipsen, have developed preparations of rhIGF-1 (Mecasermin and Increlex). Mecasermin, is the principal mediator of the somatotropic effects of human growth hormone and is used to treat growth failure in children and adolescents with severe primary insulin-like growth factor-1 deficiency.

Is rhIGF-1 the Anabolic Agent to Use?

Reviews of rhGH/rhIGF-1 combinations in GH resistance are more positive than either alone, but the literature on their combined use in sports is limited. Tests for detecting rhGH use are reaching their zenith and consequently athletes are doping with rhIGF-1. IGF-1 stimulates skeletal muscle protein synthesis, which makes it as attractive as rhGH as a doping agent. The effects of rhIGF-1 on physical exercise and anthropometry is being investigated, based on similar measurement of markers as rhGH action, with the hope of being available in time for the 2012 Olympics [45]. No athlete has yet tested positive for rhIGF. Personal communications with athletes by the authors in unpublished research has identified the extent of use in sports. Athletes believe that the combination is more powerful than double of either alone and lower doses of either will limit detection.

HISTORY OF INSULIN

Sir Edward Schafer, Professor of Physiology in Edinburgh, appears to have been the first to name insulin and describe its actions in 1913 [46]. Insulin was subsequently discovered by Banting and Best in 1921. The first patient was treated a year later in 1922. Professors Baylis and Starling at University College, London, had previously described "secretin" as the first hormone to be isolated and characterized. They had coined the term "hormones" to describe the class of substance produced in one part of the body and acting elsewhere. Schafer preferred his own term, "insuline," which was based on terms used at the time to describe actions of drugs, with excitatory and inhibitory action. His description of how he thought the hypothetical substance "insulin" acted in the body is remarkable because the passage of time has shown him to be very accurate [8].

Physiology of Insulin

Insulin is a two chain (30 & 21 amino-acids, molecular weight 5808 daltons) polypeptide hormone synthesised and secreted by the Beta-cells of the islets of Langerhans in the pancreas gland. Insulin acts in a stimulatory and an inhibitory manner [46]. It stimulates the translocation of glucose transporters ('Glut 4') from the cytoplasm of muscle and adipose tissue to the cell membrane. This increases the rate of glucose uptake to values greater than in the basal state without insulin, shown in isolated adipocytes from rats and is illustrated in figure 1. Insulin exhibits both inhibitory and excitatory actions via the same receptor. In experiments carried out on rat adipose tissue, in vitro insulin simultaneously inhibits lipolysis (the release of glycerol from stored triglyceride) and stimulates lipogenesis (formation of stored triglyceride from glucose).

Thus its anabolic action is due to two mechanisms working synergistically [47].

In *Figure 1*, it can be seen that simultaneously with insulin's excitatory effect in stimulating lipogenesis it also exhibits an inhibitory effect in preventing glycerol release. It is this inhibitory effect on lipolysis (and also glycolysis, gluconeogenesis, ketogenesis and proteolysis) that accounts for most of insulin's physiological effects in vivo in man. The inhibitory effects are also responsible for insulin's net anabolic actions.

The introduction of dynamic tracer studies enabled the identification of insulin's action in vivo in man [48]. Glucose infusion labelled with either radioactive or stable isotopes allowed the accurate measure of the rates of glucose production and rates of glucose utilisation in the circulating blood. Insulin is not needed for glucose uptake and utilisation in man i.e. glucose uptake is not totally insulin dependent.

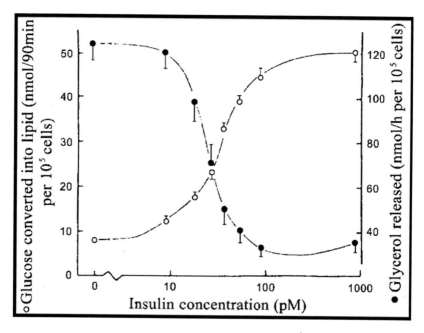

Figure 1. The anabolic actions of insulin (Adapted from Thomas *et al.* 1979) [47].

However, insulin increases glucose metabolism more through reducing FFA and ketone levels more than it does through recruiting more glucose transporters into the muscle cell membrane. Insulin does have a direct action recruiting more glucose transporters into muscle cell membranes. This facilitates glucose uptake which is reflected as an increase in the metabolic clearance rate (MCR) of glucose [48]. These protein carriers are known as glucose 'transporters'. In the case of glucose (GLUTs) there are at least six types and they tend to be tissue-specific. In the case of muscle the transporter is called 'Glut 4'. It is normally present in excess in the cell membrane even in the absence of insulin and is not rate limiting for glucose entry into the cell. Glucose transport into the cell is mainly determined by the concentration gradient between the extracellular fluid and the intracellular 'free' glucose. 'Free' glucose is very low inside the cell as it is immediately phosphorylated. Insulin recruits more transporters into the cell membrane from an intracellular pool. This increases the rate of glucose entry for a given glucose concentration and this is reflected in vivo by an increase in the MCR of glucose [49].

Is Insulin the Anabolic Agent to Use?

Insulin inhibits lipolysis and stimulates lipogenesis over the same concentration range and mediated by the same receptor [47]. Hill and Milner (1985)[50] have shown that insulin is a potent mitogen for many cell types in vitro. Sato and colleagues, (1986) [51] demonstrated that an increase in glucose metabolism to exogenous insulin in athletes (determined by euglycaemic insulin-clamp technique) was significantly higher than controls. $\dot{V}$ O$_2$peak was also significantly increased after one month's physical training. His data showed that tissue sensitivity to physiological hyper-insulinaemia was 46% higher in trained athletes and that physical training improved insulin sensitivity and lipid metabolism. Insulin has effects on protein synthesis and breakdown in muscle, at concentrations seen after meals [52]. Protein synthesis is not performed by insulin but by its regulation of IGF-1 and GH ([53] Its anabolic actions are believed to improve performance, by increasing protein synthesis [54;55] and inhibiting protein catabolism and enhancing transport of selected amino acids in human skeletal muscle [56]. The work of Bonadonna and colleagues (1993) [54] demonstrated that physiological hyper-insulinaemia stimulates the activity of amino acid transport in human skeletal muscle, thereby stimulating protein synthesis.

Hyper-aminoacidaemia specifically stimulates muscle protein synthesis and that even in the presence of hyper-aminoacidaemia insulin improves muscle protein balance, solely by inhibiting proteolysis [57]. In addition to its role in regulating glucose metabolism, insulin increases amino acid transport into cells. Its stimulation of lipogenesis, and diminished lipolysis, is one of the reasons why body builders and athletes will take rhGH in conjunction, to counteract this adverse effect, whilst optimizing protein synthesis [8].

The administration of exogenous insulin, establishes an in-vivo hyper-insulinaemic clamp, increasing muscle glycogen, before and in the recovery stages of strenuous exercise. This is believed by the athlete to increase power, strength and stamina and assist recovery. Secondly, by inhibiting muscle protein breakdown and in conjunction with a high protein/high carbohydrate diet, insulin will have the action of increasing muscle bulk, potentially improving performance.

Erythropoietin (Epo)

Erythropoietin (Epo) is a *glycoprotein hormone* (40% carbohydrate) with a Molecular wt 34 Kilodaltons (KDa) that controls *erythropoiesis*, or red blood cell production, in the *bone*. It is a *cytokine* produced by the *peritubular capillary* endothelial cells in the *kidney* and *liver*. When *exogenous* Epo is used as a *performance-enhancing drug*, it is classified as an erythropoiesis-stimulating agent (ESA). Recombinant human erythropoietin (rhEpo), darbepoetin alfa (Dpo) and methoxy polyethylene glycol-epoetin beta (PEG-Epo) are the synthetic analogues of Epo. These ESAs are commercially available for the treatment of anaemia in humans. These drugs are understood to have performance-enhancing effects on human athletes due to their powerful stimulation of red blood cell production, thereby improving delivery of oxygen to the muscle tissues. They were believed to be widely used in the 1990s in endurance *sports*. However, there was no way at that time to directly test for it, until 2000, when a test developed by Lasne and de Ceaurriz (2000) [58] based on immunoelectorphoresis and double blotting (IEF/DB), at the French national anti-doping laboratory (LNDD) and endorsed by WADA. The test detected pharmaceutical Epo by distinguishing it from the nearly identical natural hormone normally present in an athlete's urine. In 2002, at the Winter Olympic Games in Salt Lake City, *Don Catlin*, the founder and then-director of the UCLA Olympic Analytical Lab, reported finding darbepoetin alfa, a form of erythropoietin, in a test sample for the first time in sports [59]. Since 2002, Epo tests performed by U.S. sports authorities have consisted of only a urine or "direct" test. From 2006, Epo tests at the Olympics have been conducted on both blood and urine. Testing for rhEpo in urine may seem practical at first sight but appears to be a very difficult task because the amount of endogenous Epo in urine is extremely low [60].

The physiological background for testing Epo in urine is complex and the handling of Epo by the renal tubules is poorly understood. Furthermore, exercise-induced renal ischemia and the accompanying post-exercise proteinuria may affect the clearance of this peptide hormone. At present, the method officially adopted by WADA for the confirmation of rhEpo and Dpo in urine is still based on a combination of IEF/. However, the adopted monoclonal anti-*Epo* antibodies are not mono-specific. Therefore, the test can occasionally lead to the false-positive detection of rhEpo (*epoetin*-beta) in post-exercise, protein-rich urine, or in case of contamination of the sample with microorganisms [61]. A shortcoming of the current method is the lack of definitive mass spectral data for the confirmation of a positive finding. Recently, a liquid chromatography-tandem mass spectrometry (LC/MS/MS) method for the detection and confirmation of rhEpo/Dpo in equine plasma has been reported [62]. Since the introduction of the test in 2000, Epo-using athletes have altered their dosing schemes. By injecting microdoses of rhEpo, the window of detection can be reduced to as little as 12–18 hours post-injection [63].

In one study subjects were studied for seven weeks and treated with rhEpo for four weeks with two weeks of "boosting" followed by two weeks of "maintenance" and a post period of three weeks. WADA *"Laboratory A"* determined rhEpo use in all subjects during the boosting period, whereas WADA *"Laboratory B"* found no use, with one sample to be negative, and the remaining seven to be suspicious. The detection rates decreased throughout the maintenance and post period when total hemoglobin mass and exercise performance were elevated. During this period, *"Laboratory A"* found only two of 24 samples to be positive and three to be suspicious, and *"Laboratory B"* found no positive or suspicious samples. This study demonstrates a poor correlation in test results comparing two WADA-accredited laboratories. Moreover, after the initial rhEpo "boosting" period the power to detect rhEpo use during the maintenance and post periods appears minimal [64].

Another study demonstrated up to 20% of the investigated samples do not show detectable Epo (Delanghe and Joyner, 2008). However any false-positive Epo test concerns by Beullens et al., (2006) [65] have been fiercely contested as unfounded by Catlin and his working group [66, 67] based on scientific analytical rigour. Catlin's WADA-accredited laboratory has performed the IEF/DB test for rhEpo on more than 6,800 urine samples, including more than 2,600 doping control samples from athletes. They have reported nine positive cases for rhEpo; three of these have publicly confessed to using rhEpo, three have accepted penalties, the physician of a seventh has been indicted for distribution of rhEpo, and two maintained their innocence but lost on appeal.

Is rhEpo the Anabolic Agent to Use?

In 1992 exogenous Epo was shown to increase maximal aerobic power [68]. In 2010, *Floyd Landis* admitted to using performance-enhancing drugs, including Epo, throughout the majority of his career as a professional cyclist [69]. This demonstrates the difficulty in detecting doping with Epo. Exogenous Epo can often be detected in blood, due to slight difference from the endogenous protein, for example in features of *posttranslational modification* [42]. Further identification in blood is possible by indirect parameters of stimulated erythropoiesis.

Indirect blood analysis showed that high-dose, short-term rhEPO treatment resulted in a significant increase in the serum concentration of soluble transferrin receptor (sTfR) and the ratio between sTfR and ferritin, and also confirmed this using lower doses during longer term, but was not accepted by the authorities [70] The problem is that the duration of the effect on performance is greater than the duration of any hematological changes associated with rhEPO use. Once rhEPO administration is discontinued, red cell mass gradually returns to its original state and can take weeks. As a result, an open window may exist where there is no evidence of rhEPO use but where performance is enhanced [71].

In a study conducted by Birkeland et al., (2000) [71], 5,000 U of rhEPO three times weekly for four weeks was administered to ten male athletes. Packed cell volume (PCV, haematocrit) increased from $42.7 \pm 1.6\%$ to $50.8 \pm 2.0\%$ and peaked one day after cessation of treatment. There was an increase in sTfR (from 3.1 ± 0.9 to 6.3 ± 2.3 mg.L^{-1}, $P < 0.001$) and in the ratio between sTfR and ferritin (sTfR.ferritin^{-1}) (from 3.2 ± 1.6 to 11.8 ± 5.1, $P < 0.001$). The sTfR increase was significant after one week of treatment and remained so for one week post-treatment. $\dot{V}$ O_2max increased from 63.6 ± 4.5 mL.kg^{-1}.min^{-1} before to 68.1 ± 5.4 mL.kg^{-1}.min^{-1} two days post rhEPO administration (7% increase, $P = 0.001$) in the EPO group. The dangers to the exercising athlete are that the elevated PCV (haematocrit) could potentially lead to enhancement of clotting. In studies arterial systolic and diastolic blood pressure (BP) at rest remain unaltered before and after rhEPO admin. During submaximal exercise at 200 watts, corresponding to an average of approx 50% of $\dot{V}$ O$_2$max, there is a marked increase in arterial systolic BP from 177 to 191 mmHg, demonstrating increased stress on the heart during heavy strenuous and prolonged exercise [72]. During competition cycling and running the average energy turn-over is often in the range of 75-85% of $\dot{V}$ O$_2$max for long periods. Thus elevated arterial BP due to rhEPO injections could explain unexpected deaths of young cyclists, in the last decade! Within the first four years of rhEPO's introduction, this synthetic hormone was suggested to have caused over 17 athletes' deaths [73]. Sandro Donati, an Italian professor of exercise physiology suggests that, rhEPO was being used by 60-70% percent of all professional cyclists. He also claimed Italian sport's doctors were administering rhEPO to professional cyclists for large annual fees of $50,000-$100,000 [74].

CURRENT RESEARCH - A MYOSTATIN INHIBITOR (FOLLISTATIN)

Myostatin is a transforming growth factor-β (TGF-β) family member that plays an essential role in regulating skeletal muscle growth. It acts as a negative regulator of skeletal muscle mass. Pharmacological agents capable of blocking myostatin activity may have applications for promoting muscle growth in human disease. Follistatin, also known as activin-binding protein is a peptide hormone, in humans, encoded by the FST *gene*. Follistatin is an *autocrine glycoprotein* that is expressed in nearly all tissues. It is part of the inhibin-activin-follistatin axis and is produced by folliculostellate (FS) cells of the anterior pituitary. In the tissues activin has a strong role in *cellular proliferation*, thereby making follistatin the safeguard against uncontrolled cellular proliferation and also allowing it to function as an instrument of *cellular differentiation*. Both of these roles are vital in tissue rebuilding and repair.

Follistatin has been assessed for its role in regulation of muscle growth in mice, as an antagonist to *myostatin*. Lee & McPherron (2001) [75] demonstrated that inhibition of myostatin, either by genetic elimination *(knockout mice)* or by increasing the amount of follistatin, resulted in greatly increased muscle mass. Mice that lack the gene that makes myostatin have roughly twice the amount of body muscle as normal. But mice without myostatin that also overproduce follistatin have about four times as much muscle as normal mice [76]. In 2009, research with *macaque* monkeys [77] has demonstrated that regulating follistatin via *gene therapy* also resulted in muscle growth and increases in strength Such research paves the way for future control of disease states, but the application for the use of a myostatin inhibitor in sport is all too evident.

Availability of rhGH, rhIGF, Insulin and Follistatin

Unscrupulous individuals purchase prescription rhGH and insulin from benefit agency patients. Some are from the parents of children with growth disorders, who are being deprived of their medicine (personal communications). Bodybuilders and athletes have been known to purchase insulin from insulin dependent diabetics, who get free "pen-fills" paid for by the NHS. Despite insulin being dangerous in overdose, it is a pharmacy medicine and can be purchased over the counter, from a "friendly" pharmacist for the athlete's "diabetic dog". Another source is the black market, where dealers are distributing potentially counterfeit products masquerading as rhGH. Counterfeit products include mannitol and human chorionic gonadotrphin (HCG). Mannitol, a sugar alcohol, will have no effect, but is cheap. HCG is a polypeptide glycoprotein hormone of 244 *amino* with a *molecular mass* of 36.7 Kda, produced by the female placenta, and has the same action as pituitary luteinising hormone (LH) and has been used by bodybuilders in an attempt to prevent testicular atrophy during pronged AAS use. It restores testicular size as well as normal testosterone production. It has some side-effects that mimic rhGH, which make it popular with counterfeiters, but no performance enhancement. The internet has encouraged the abuse of very expensive designer drugs, particularly rhGH, rhIGF and rhEPO, resulting in an increase in importation for personal use.

CONCLUSION

The Internet would appear to be the virtual superstore for the budding doping elite athlete of the future. The provenance of products purchased from the "other side of the globe" will always be in doubt and as a consequence, Pandora's box will always be half open [41]. Interestingly, muscle-growth genes and mRNA expression can be increased and myostatin can be down regulated following essential amino acids ingestion and an anabolic stimulus [78].

REFERENCES

[1]   Li, CH; Evans, HM; Simpson; ME. Isolation and properties of the anterior hypophyseal growth hormone. *J Biol Chem*, 1945 159, 353–366.

[2]   Fryklund, L. Current research on recombinant human *Acta Paediatr Scand Suppl*, 1986 325, 85-89.

[3]   Kaplan, SL; Underwood, LE; August, GP; Bell, JJ; Blethen, SL; Blizzard, RM; Brown, DR; Foley, TP; Hintz, RL; Hopwood, NJ. Clinical studies with recombinant-DNA-derived methionyl human growth hormone in growth hormone deficient children. *Lancet*, 1986 29, 697-700.

[4]   Holt, RIG; Sonksen, PH. Growth hormone, IGF-I and insulin and their abuse in sport. *British Journal of Pharmacology*, 2008 154, 542–546.

[5]   Bachl, N; Derman, W; Engebretsen, L; Goldspink, G; Kinzlbauer, M; Tschan, H; Volpi, P; Venter, D; Wessner, B. Therapeutic use of growth factors in the musculoskeletal system in sports-related injuries. *J Sports Med Phys Fitness,* 2009 49, 346-357.

[6]   Duchaine, D. *Underground Steroid Handbook*, 1st ed. California: HLR Technical Books, 1982 84.

[7]   Wallace, JD; Cuneo, RC; Lundberg, PA; Rosen, T; Jorgensen, JOL; Longobardi, S; Keay, N; Sacca, L; Christiansen, JS; Bengtsson, B-A; Sonksen, PH. Responses of markers of bone and collagen turnover to exercise, growth hormone (GH) administration and GH withdrawal in trained adult males. *J Clin Endocrinol Metab*, 2000 85, 124–133.

[8]   Sonksen, PH. Insulin, growth hormone and sport. *J Endocrinol*, 2001 170, 13-25.

[9]   Konrad, C; Schupfer, G; Wietlisbach, M; Gerber, H. Insulin as an anabolic: hypoglycaemia in the bodybuilding world. *Anaesthesiol Intensivmed Schmerzther*, 1998 33, 461-463.

[10] Evans, PJ; Lynch, RM. Insulin as a drug of abuse in body building. *Br J Sports Med*, 2003 37, 356-357.

[11] Dawson, RT. Drugs in Sport. The role of the physician. *Journal of Endocrinology*, 2001 170, 55-61.

[12] Grace, FM; Baker, JS; Davies, B. Anabolic Androgenic Steroid (AAS) Use in Recreational Gym Users- A regional sample of the Mid-Glamorgan area. *J Substance Use*, 2001 12, 145-153.

[13] Graham, MR; Baker, JS; Davies, B. "Steroid" and prescription medicine abuse in the health and fitness community; a regional study. *Eur J Intern Med*, 2006 17, 479-484.

[14] (*http://www.telegraph.co.uk/sport/othersports/drugsinsport/7293877.html.*)

[15] (*http://www.cyclingweekly.co.uk/news/latest/519647.html*

[16] Baumann G. Growth hormone heterogeneity: genes, isohormones, variants, and binding proteins. *Endocr Rev*, 1991 12, 424–449.

[17] Wu, Z; Bidlingmaier, M; Dall, R; Strasburger, CJ. Detection of doping with human growth hormone. *Lancet* 1999 353, 895.

[18] Melmed, S. Medical progress: Acromegaly. *N Engl J Med*, 2006 14, 2558-2573.

[19] Kojima, M; Hosoda, H; Date, Y; Nakazato, M; Matsuo, H; Kangawa, K. Ghrelin is a growth-hormone-releasing acylated peptide from stomach. *Nature*, 1999 9, 656-660.

[20] Iranmanesh, A; Lizarralde, G; Velduis, JD. Age and relative adiposity are specific negative determinants of the frequency and amplitude of growth hormone secretory bursts and the half-life of endogenous GH in healthy men. *J Clin Endocrinol Metab*, 1991 73, 1081-1088.

[21] Brown, RJ; Adams, JJ; Pelekanos, RA; Wan, Y; McKinstry, WJ; Palethorpe, K; Seeber, RM; Monks, TA; Eidne, KA; Parker, MW; Waters, MJ. Model for growth hormone receptor activation based on subunit rotation within a receptor dimer. *Nat Struct Mol Biol*, 2005 12, 814-821.

[22] Argetsinger, LS; Campbell, GS; Yang, X; Witthuhn, BA; Silvennoinen, O; Ihle, JN; Carter-Su, C. Identification of JAK2 as a growth hormone receptor-associated tyrosine kinase. *Cell*, 1993 237-244.

[23] Le Roith, D; Scavo, L; Butler, A. What is the role of circulating IGF-I? *Trends Endocrinol Metab*, 2001 12, 48-52.

[24] O'Reilly, KE; Rojo, F; She, QB; Solit, D; Mills, GB; Smith, D; Lane, H; Hofmann, F; Hicklin, DJ; Ludwig, DL; Baselga, J; Rosen, N. mTOR inhibition induces upstream receptor tyrosine kinase signaling and activates *Akt Cancer Res*, 2006 66, 1500-1508.

[25] Milani, D; Carmichael, JD; Welkowitz, J; Ferris, S; Reitz, RE Variability and reliability of single serum IGF-I measurements: impact

on determining predictability of risk ratios in disease development. *J Clin Endocrinol Metab*, 2004 89, 2271-2274.

[26] Velloso, C, Aperghis, M, Godfrey, R, et al. The effects of two weeks recombinant growth hormone administration on the response of IGF-I and PIIIP to a single bout of high intensity resistance exercise in resistance trained young men. *Communication to the Physiological Society, University College London, Conference Proceedings*, 2006, C48.

[27] Mauras, N; Attie, KM; Reiter, EO; Saenger, P; Baptista, J. High dose recombinant human growth hormone (GH) treatment of GH-deficient patients in puberty increases near-final height: a randomized, multicenter trial. Genentech, Inc., Cooperative Study Group. *J Clin Endocrinol Metab*, 2000 85, 3653-3660.

[28] Stabler, B; Turner, JR; Girdler, SS; Light KC, Underwood LE. Reactivity to stress and psychological adjustment in adults with pituitary insufficiency. *Clin Endocrinol (Oxf)*, 1992 6, 467-473.

[29] Graham, MR; Davies, B; Kicman, A; Cowan, D; Hullin, D; Baker, JS. Recombinant human *Curr Neurovasc Res*, 2007 4, 9-18.

[30] Crist, DM; Peake, GT; Egan, PA; Waters, DL. Body composition response to exogenous GH during training in highly conditioned adults. *J Appl Physiol*, 1988 65, 579-584.

[31] Fryburg, DA; Gelfand, RA; Barrett, EJ. Growth hormone acutely stimulates forearm muscle protein synthesis in normal humans. *Am J Physiol*, 1991 260, 499–504.

[32] Lange, KH; Andersen, JL; Beyer, N; Isaksson, F; Larsson, B; Rasmussen, MH; Juul, A; Bülow, J; Kjaer, M. GH admin changes myosin heavy chain isoforms in skeletal muscle but does not augment muscle strength or hypertrophy, either alone or combined with resistance exercise training in healthy elderly men. *J Clin Endocrinol Metab*, 2002 87, 513–23.

[33] Healy, ML; Gibney, J; Russell-Jones, DL; Pentecost, C; Croos, P; Sönksen, PH; Umpleby, AM. High Dose Growth Hormone Exerts an Anabolic Effect at Rest and during Exercise in Endurance-Trained Athletes. *J Clin Endocrinol Metab*, 2003 11, 5221-5226.

[34] Nørrelund, H; Nair, KS; Nielsen, S; Frystyk, J; Ivarsen, P; Jørgensen, JO; Christiansen, JS; Møller, N. The Decisive Role of Free Fatty Acids for Protein Conservation during Fasting in Humans with and without Growth Hormone. *J Clin Endocrinol Metab*, 2003 88, 4371-4378.

[35] Ehrnborg, C; Ellegard, L; Bosaeus, I; Bengtsson, BA; Rosen, T. Supraphysiological growth hormone: less fat, more extracellular fluid but uncertain effects on muscles in healthy, active young adults. *Clin Endocrinol (Oxf)*, 2005 62, 449-457.

[36] Healy, ML; Gibney, J; Pentecost, C; Croos, P; Russell-Jones, DL; Sönksen, PH; Umpleby, AM. Effects of High-Dose Growth Hormone on Glucose and Glycerol Metabolism at Rest and during Exercise in Endurance-Trained Athletes. *J Clin Endocrinol Metab*, 2006 91, 320-327.

[37] Liu, W; Thomas, SG; Asa, SL; Gonzalez-Cadavid, N; Bhasin, S; Ezzat S. Myostatin Is a Skeletal Muscle Target of Growth Hormone Anabolic Action. *J Clin Endocrinol Metab*, 2003 88, 5490-5496.

[38] Wallace, JD; Cuneo, RC; Baxter, R; Orskov, H; Keay, N; Pentecost, C; Dall, R; Rosen, T; Jorgensen, JO; Cittadini, A; Longobardi, S; Sacca, L; Christiansen, JS, Bengtsson, B-A; Sonksen, PH. Responses of the growth hormone (GH) and insulin-like growth factor axis to exercise, GH administration, and GH withdrawal in trained adult males: a potential test for GH abuse in sport. *J Clin Endocrinol Metab*, 1999 84, 3591–3601.

[39] Graham, MR; Baker, JS; Evans, P; Kicman, A; Cowan, D; Hullin, D; Thomas, N; Davies, B. Physical effects of short term rhGH administration in abstinent steroid dependency. *Hormone Research*, 2008 69, 343-354.

[40] Graham, MR; Baker, JS; Evans, P; Hullin, D; Thomas, NE; Davies, B. Potential benefits *Growth Horm IGF Res*, 2009a 19, 300-307.

[41] Graham, MR; Ryan, P; Baker, JS; Davies, B; Thomas, NE; Cooper, SM; Evans, P; Easmon, S; Walker, CJ; Cowan, D; Kicman, AT. Counterfeiting in performance- and image *Drug Test. Anal.*, 2009b 1, 135-1342.

[42] Yu, NH; Ho, EN; Wan, TS; Wong, AS. Doping control analysis of recombinant human *Anal Bioanal Chem*, 2010 396, 2513-2521.

[43] Powrie, JK; Bassett, EE; Rosen, T; Jørgensen, JO; Napoli, R; Sacca, L; Christiansen, JS; Bengtsson, BA; Sönksen, PH. Detection of growth hormone abuse in sport. On behalf of the GH-2000 Project study group. *Growth Horm IGF Res*, 2007 17, 220-226.

[44] Mauras, N; Haymond, MW. Are the metabolic effects of GH and IGF-I separable. *Growth Hormone and IGF Research*, 2005 15, 19-27.

[45] Guha, N; Sönksen, PH; Holt, RI. IGF-I abuse in sport: current knowledge and future prospects for detection. *Growth Horm IGF Res*, 2009 19, 408-4011.

[46] Schafer, E. *The Endocrine Organs*. London: Longman, Green & Co, 1916

[47] Thomas, SHL; Wisher, MH; Brandenburg, D; Sonksen, PH. Insulin action on Adipocytes. Evidence that the anti-lipolytic and lipogenic effects of insulin are medicated by the same receptor. *Biochem J*, 1979 184, 355-360.

[48] Sonksen, PH; Sonksen, J. Insulin: Understanding its action in health and disease. *British Journal of Anaesthesia*, 2000 85, 69-79.

[49] Boroujerdi, MA; Umpleby, AM; Jones, RH; Sonksen, PH. A simulation model for glucose kinetics and estimates of glucose utilization rate in type I diabetic patients. *Am J Physiol*. 1995 268, 766-774.

[50] Hill, DJ; Milner, RDG. Insulin as a Growth Factor. *Paediatr Res*, 1985 19, 879-886.

[51] Sato, Y; Hayamizu, S; Yamamoto, C; Ohkuwa, Y; Yamanouchi, K; Sakamoto, N. Improved insulin sensitivity in carbohydrate and lipid metabolism after physical training. Int. *J Sports Med*, 1986 7, 307-310.

[52] Bennet, WM; Connacher, AA; Scrimgeour, CM; Smith, K; Rennie, MJ. Increase in anterior tibialis muscle protein synthesis in healthy man during mixed amino acid infusion: studies of incorporation of $[1-^{13}C]$ leucine. *Clin Sci*, 1989 76, 447–454.

[53] Bennet, WM; Connacher, AA; Scrimgeour, CM; Jung, RT; Rennie, MJ. Euglycaemic hyperinsulinaemia augments amino acid uptake by human leg tissues during hyperaminoacidaemia. *Am J Physiol*, 1990 259, 185-194.

[54] Bonadonna, RC; Saccomani, MP; Cobelli, C; Defronzo, RA. Effect of Insulin on System A Amino Acid Transport in Human Skeletal Muscle. *J Clin Invest*, 1993 91, 514-521.

[55] Kimball, SR; Vary, TC; Jefferson, LS. Regulation of protein synthesis by insulin. *Ann Rev Physiol*, 1994 56, 321-348.

[56] Biolo, G; Fleming, RYD; Wolfe, RD. Physiologic Hyperinsulinaemia Stimulates Protein Synthesis and Enhances Transport of Selected Amino Acids in Human Skeletal Muscle. *J Clin Invest*, 1995 95, 811-819.

[57] Fryburg, DA; Jahn, LA; Hill, SA; Oliveras, DM; Barrett, EJ. Insulin and Insulin-like Growth Factor-I enhance human skeletal muscle protein anabolism during hyperaminoacidaemia by different mechanisms. *J Clin Invest*, 1995 96, 1722-1729.

[58] Lasne, F; de Ceaurriz, J. Recombinant erythropoietin in urine. *Nature*, 2000 405, 635.

[59] Catlin, DH; Breidbach, A; Elliott, S; Glaspy, J. Effects of oral androstenedione administration on serum *J Clin Endocrinol Metab*, 2002 87, 5449-5454.

[60] Franke, WW; Heid, H. Pitfalls, errors and risks of false-positive results in urinary EPO drug tests. *Clin Chim Acta*, 2006 373, 189–190.

[61] Delanghe, JR; Joyner, MJ. Testing for recombinant human *J Appl Physiol*, 2008 105, 395-396.

[62] Guan, F; Uboh, CE; Soma, LR; Birks, E; Chen, J; You, Y; Rudy, J; Li, X. Differentiation and identification *Anal Chem*, 2008 80, 3811-3817.

[63] Ashenden, M; Varlet-Marie, E; Lasne, F; Audran, M. The effects of microdose recombinant human erythropoietin regimens in athletes. *Haematologica, 2006* 91, 1143–1144.

[64] Lundby, C; Achman-Andersen, NJ; Thomsen, JJ; Norgaard, AM; Robach, P. Testing for recombinant human *J Appl Physiol*, 2008 105, 417-419.

[65] Beullens, M; Delanghe, JR; Bollen, M. False-positive detection of recombinant human erythropoietin in urine following strenuous physical exercise. *Blood*, 2006 107, 4711-4713.

[66] Catlin, D; Green, G; Sekera, M; Scott, P; Starcevic, B. False-positive Epo test concerns unfounded. *Blood*, 2006 108, 1779-17780.

[67] Catlin, D; Nissen-Lie, G; Howe, C; Pascual, JA; Lasne, F; Saugy, M. Harmonization of the method for the identification of epoetin alfa and beta (rEPO) and darbepoetin alfa (NESP) by IEF-double blotting and chemiluminescent detection. *WADA Technical Document TD2007EPO*. Available at *http://www.wada-ama.org/rtecontent/document/td2007epo_en.pdf*.

[68] Ekblom, B; Berglund B. Effect of rhEPO admin on maximal aerobic power in man. *Medicine & Science in Sports & Exercise*, 1991; 1: 125-130.

[69] (*http://www.cyclingweekly.co.uk/news/latest/519647.html*

[70] Audran, M; Gareau, R; Matecki, S; Durand, F; Chenard, C; Sicart, MT; Marion, B; Bressolle, F. Effects of erythropoietin *Med Sci Sports Exerc*, 1999 31, 639-645.

[71] Birkeland, KI; Stray-Gundersen, J; Hemmersbach, P; Hallen, J; Haug, E; Bahr, R. Effect of rhEPO administration on serum levels of sTfR and cycling performance. *Med Sci Sports Exerc*, 2000 32, 1238-1243.

[72] Berglund, B; Ekblom, B. Effect of rhEPO treatment on BP and haematological parameters in healthy males. *Journal of Internal Medicine*, 1991 229, 125-130.

[73] Ramotar, J. Cyclists' deaths linked to erythropoietin? *Physician and Sports Medicine*, 1990 18, 48-49.

[74] Martin, DT; Ashenden, M; Parisotto, R; Pyne, D; Hahn, AG. Blood testing for professional cyclists: what's a fair hematocrit limit? *Sportscience News*, 1997   http://www.sportsci.org/news/news9703 /AISblood.html

[75] Lee, SJ; McPherron, AC. Regulation of myostatin activity and muscle growth *Proc Natl Acad Sci USA*, 2001 98, 9306-9311.

[76] 'Mighty mice' made *mightier http://www.eurekalert.org/pub_releases /2007-08/jhmi-mm082407.php.*

[77] "Success Boosting Monkey Muscle Could Help Humans" *http://www.npr.org/templates/story/story.php?storyId=120316010*

[78] Drummond, MJ; Glynn, EL; Fry, CS; Dhanani, S; Volpi, E; Rasmussen, BB. Essential amino acids increase microRNA-499, -208b, and -23a and downregulate myostatin and myocyte enhancer factor 2C mRNA expression in human skeletal muscle. *J Nutr*, 2009 139, 2279-2284.

INDEX

J

K

L

M

Q

R

S